RUN HEALTHY, RUN STRONG

RUN HEALTHY, RUN STRONG

Dr. Steve Smith's Guide
to Injury Prevention
& Treatment for Runners

STEVEN L. SMITH, D.C.

PACERS
PRESS

Pacers Press
131 N. El Molino Ave., Pasadena, CA 91101
First Edition: February 2013.

Author photograph by Bill Youngblood.
Illustrations Mary Ann Zapalac.
Book design and typesetting by Ashlee Goodwin, Hive Creative.

Please visit our website
RUNHEALTHYRUNSTRONG.COM

*This book is dedicated to my wife, Robin,
whose continuous flow of intense admiration
makes all things possible. She has been at my side
on all the long hard days, weathered the burdens
of defeat and shared great victories with me.
This book is one of those victories.*

CONTENTS

INTRODUCTION

The Road to Healthy Running   15

CHAPTER 1

The Changing Face of Running   21
   and the Second Running Boom

CHAPTER 2

Rest: The Magical Miracle Cure for Almost Any Injury   25

CHAPTER 3

Preventing & Treating Common Injuries
   Illiotibial Band Syndrome   29
   The Knee   40
   Leg Injuries   44
   Ankle Injuries   46
   Foot Injuries   50
   Back Problems   59

CHAPTER 4

Safety for Runners
   Sensory Perception   65
   Traffic   67
   Choosing a Safe Running Route   69
   Weather   72
   Crime and Other Dangers   80

CHAPTER 5

A Matter of Heart   85

CHAPTER 6

Cross-Training 93

CHAPTER 7

ChiRunning 99

CHAPTER 8

Running Shoes 103

CHAPTER 9

Ankle/Calf/Shin/Achilles Exercises

Shin Strengthening 1	117
Shin Strengthening 2	118
Heavy Load Eccentric Contraction	119
Achilles Press	120

ITB Exercises

TheraBand Crab Walk	121
Side-lying Hip Abduction	122
Lying Side Plank	123
Hip Hike	124

Knee/Quad Exercises

Sumo Walk	125
One Legged Plie	126
Walking Lunge	127
Knee Drive	128
Three Way Step Down	129
Four Way Cross	130
Supine Quad Press	132
Groucho	133

Core Exercises
   Prone Plank   134
   Single Straight Leg Raise   135
   V-Sit   136
   One Leg V-Sit   137

Gluteal Exercises
   Butt Press   138
   Bridging   139
   Wrestler's Bridge   140
   Donkey Kicks   141
   Butt Blaster   142

Hip and Groin Exercises
   Fire Buckets   143
   Three Point Touch   144
   Hip Adductor   145

Plyometrics
   Rocket Jumps   146
   Lunge Spring   147
   Bounding   148
   Frog Jump   149
   Speed Skater   150
   Side Hurdle   151

Stretches
   Lower Calf   152
   Upper Calf   153
   Hamstring   154
   Quad/Shin Double Stretch   155
   Illiotibial Band   156

Stretches continued

Scissor Kick   157

Side Scissors   158

Hip   159

Upper Chest   160

Lower Chest   161

CHAPTER 10

Final Thoughts   163

RUNNING COMMENTARIES

Heavy Usage: Why Runners Court the Risk of Injury   38

A Special Note About Cyclists   70

Why We Run in the Rain   74

Why It's Smart to Run With a Partner or Group   82

How Often Should You Replace Running Shoes?   104

On Running Barefoot   108

Should You Stretch Before or After a Run?   113

Index   166

ACKNOWLEDGMENTS

My thanks to all the volunteers at the San Gabriel Leukemia Team-in-Training for inviting me to be their instructor on healthy running, especially coaches Kylie Akers, Van and Virginia Garnet and Dave Hagen. You are incredibly effective at helping more people than you even know.

My thanks to ChiRunning instructor and friend, Kathy Greist. I appreciate the knowledge and skill you've brought me.

My thanks to Peter Van Gansen, owner of Run with Us, the finest running store I know of, and his amazing staff. Your place has become a focal point of our running community. I thank you for that, and for your friendship.

My thanks to Ashlee Goodwin, book designer extraordinaire, for your talent, wisdom and friendship.

Finally, my thanks to all the Pasadena Pacers, particularly Dave McCarthy who does such a magnificent job welcoming and training our newest members (and thus, enabling me to run); Ezra Weiss who brings great humor and the graceful spirit of Tai Chi to our warm-up program; Hilda Xicara and Wende Lee, two of our most enthusiastic and dedicated coaches.

SPECIAL THANKS

To my friend and writing partner,
Leslie Lindeman,
without whose contribution
this book would not be all that it is.

"I believe we can raise the health and spirit of mankind through fitness."

—STEVE SMITH
JUNE 6, 1996

*If you run, you are
a runner...There
is no test to pass,
no license to earn, no
membership card to
get. You just run.*

JOHN BINGHAM

INTRODUCTION

The Road to Healthy Running

SINCE 1979 I've had a Chiropractic practice based largely on treating runners. The worst thing about my job is seeing grown men cry. Women also. If you're a runner it could happen to you. In fact, the odds are, it will.

Maybe you've signed up for a race. Maybe you are in the middle of a training program. You've spent money, planned to take time off from work, and you've set goals. Or maybe you're not training for a particular race; you're just excited to be running outside after a long winter. Running makes you happy. Running is your fix.

But then, without warning, some part of your body begins to hurt. At first it's just a little sore, but pretty soon it's painful, and suddenly it's clear: you can't run.

Just like that, the fun is gone. And the fitness, the camaraderie, and the emotional release are gone with it.

Soon after, someone in my profession is handing you a diagnosis and telling you that you can't run for weeks or maybe months. You can't be out there with your friends training this weekend, you won't be able to make the race next month—in effect, you're off the team.

It reminds you of your childhood when someone told you you couldn't go out for recess. Or maybe a time when you didn't get invited to the big party. "I'm sorry, but you have to stop running." The words are hard to speak and worse to hear. It might sound extreme, but they break hearts. I've seen people cry so often that I know to have tissues close at hand before I deliver the news.

Studies tell us that running has a high incidence of injury, as high as 79%, and indications are that injuries happen most often to beginning runners. If you've been running for several years, you don't need to read the studies. You've probably gone through your share of aches and strains. You've seen your friends sidelined, too.

But here's the good news. It doesn't have to be this way. Studies also show that up to 60% of running injuries are avoidable. In my experience, we can do even better than that.

That's why I've written this book. From decades treating every common runner's injury hundreds of times, and most of the exotic ones several times as well, I've learned a few simple ways of approaching running that can keep the injuries away and minimize them when they do occur. In these pages you will find the best information I've been able to bring together in one place that will help you run healthy, strong and injury-free.

I encourage you to take action with the simple strategies for running healthy you will find here. Enjoy our sport, stay on the team, and I will see you out on the road.

—Dr. Smith

PASADENA PACERS FOUNDER STEVE SMITH RUNS WITH A FELLOW PACER DURING SATURDAY MORNING PRACTICE AT THE PASADENA ROSE BOWL.

PHOTO SEAN SMITH

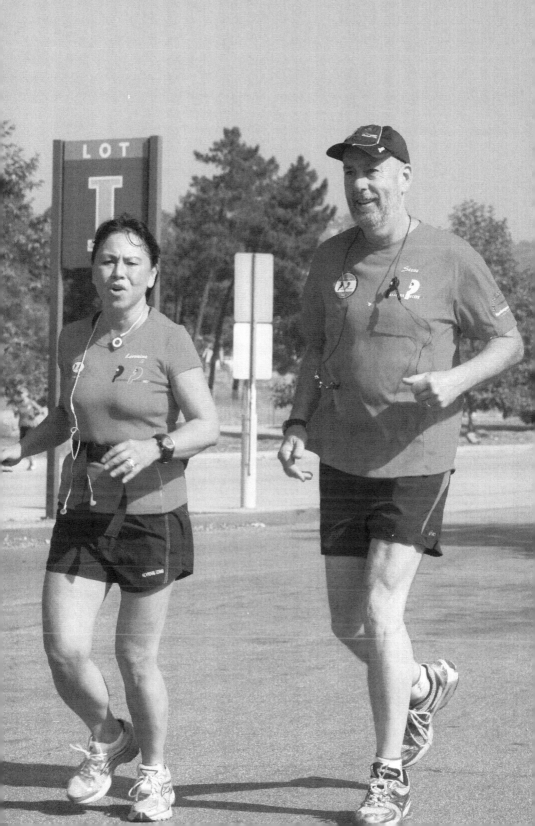

We may train or peak
for a certain race,
but running is
a lifetime sport.

ALBERTO SALAZAR

CHAPTER 1

The Changing Face of Running and the Second Running Boom

RUNNING IS MORE popular than ever. In the United States there are 16 million "hard-core" runners, meaning those of us who run more than 100 times a year. There are also 43 million American runners—more than 10 percent of the entire population—meaning those of us who run at least once in a year.

In 2009, for the first time ever, the number of runners who completed a road race cracked the 10 million mark. That included almost half a million people who finished a marathon and more than 1 million who completed half-marathons. All those numbers constitute records and they tell us we are in the middle of the second running boom in U.S. history and that it's much bigger than the first one which occurred some 40 years ago.

But this may be the most interesting development. Twenty years ago running was a man's sport. Men outnumbered women in road races by nearly 4 to 1. But today, 53 percent of runners crossing the finish line in road races are women. As running grows rapidly in popularity the biggest joiners by far are women.

I'm not surprised. These developments are written in our DNA.

The physical act of running turns on the cerebellum, the primordial section of the brain that still works the same way it did way back when we were all hunters and gatherers. As primitive people, we moved together, worked together and lived or died together.

Running also activates the thinking and emotional sections of the brain. As cavemen chasing a mastodon, our prefrontal cortexes governed mental processing, such as how we moved into position and the way we aimed our spears.

The prefrontal cortex was also the doorway to experiencing and understanding emotions. It took big emotions like aggression in order to kill animals bigger than we were. But we also needed to understand subtle feelings such as the mood of our brother cavemen, because knowing whether Og was going to zig or zag at a crucial moment could lead to a dead mastodon or a dead cavemen.

As the tribe moved, its members became one. Whether moving slowly through a patch of berries or running down prey, the feeling of community became part of who we were. There was a sense of well-being that came from being part of the group.

These feelings have remained part of the human experience throughout the chain of evolution and are alive in us today.

When the first running boom took off in the 1970s, running was seen as an individual sport. Our picture was of the iconic runner racing alone over great distances. Indeed, the marathon takes its name from the legend of the Greek messenger, Pheidippides, who ran 26 miles from Marathon to Athens to deliver word that Greece had defeated the Persians, and then collapsed and died on the spot.

Forty years ago we thought running was not for everyone. People who ran races trained by themselves and raced alone. They were a little extreme. To run a marathon you had to be crazy. At least that was the perception. What we were learning in those days—actually re-learning—was how good running is for us. We were rediscovering running one runner at a time.

Today, we are rediscovering in huge numbers that running is for everyone. It awakens deep, even ancient, feelings of physical and emotional well-being. The first high we experience is the classic "runner's high," that physical rush that comes when the endorphins are released and we feel like we can go forever, that everything is right with the world and anything is possible.

But the second "runner's high," comes from connecting with the group. I get emails every day from members of our runners club, the Pasadena Pacers, crediting the group with helping them successfully run a race, recover from an injury or find their place in a sport that is changing their lives. I never thought the Pacers would become a group that supports people to restore their health or raise it to levels they hadn't thought possible. It never occurred to me that a runner's group could help people overcome personal challenges and achieve their life's goals.

But after many years of realizing that the Pacers truly do help people accomplish all these things, I understand why so many races are filled to capacity, and that their numbers are limited only by how many people city streets can hold.

My wife, Robin, and I were in San Francisco for the marathon and half-marathon last summer, and we were out walking with a group of Pacers after dinner. The race was still hours away but the city was alive with the excitement of what the morning would bring. The police were closing streets. Volunteers were setting up aid stations. Everywhere you looked you saw people in warm-up jackets and running shoes. We could feel the energy moving through the city and I knew it was because of all the people. Suddenly, Gary, a friend of mine, turned to me and with the enthusiasm of a little kid, said, "It's so great to be with everyone!"

That's the story of the second running boom. "It's great to be with everyone." It's great to play. It's great to be part of the team.

We've made the leap from realizing that running is good for me to experiencing that running is good for us. We've gone from seeing running as an effective and fulfilling form of exercise, to understanding and benefiting from the joys of person-to-person interaction and the power of the group.

Running makes us strong individually, but running with the team makes us even stronger. As the Rudyard Kipling saying goes, "The strength of the pack is the wolf, and the strength of the wolf is the pack."

Running will always have its challenges—from heat to biting cold, wind, rain, hills, distance and fatigue—but when our will flags, we turn to each other. There is an intangible boost that comes from running with a friend or a group. Somehow, each of us goes farther and faster than we could have if we were set apart, each on his own course.

The joys and benefits of the group are why running shuts down major city streets every weekend. Team sports draw more spectators but running is unique in its ability to draw millions of participants onto such a vigorous field of play.

So I want to honor your commitment to the sport, to your own health and well-being, and if you choose, to your contributing and benefiting from a running group that can change and improve lives on the road and off.

*In running, it
doesn't matter whether
you come in first, in the
middle of the pack, or
last. You can say,
"I have finished."*

FRED LEBOW

CHAPTER 2

Rest: The Magical Miracle Cure for Almost Any Injury

REST IS THE first line of defense against most running injuries and rest is usually the first treatment option when we do come down with an injury. The smartest thing we can do when creating a training program is build in sufficient rest.

Most runners recover pretty quickly from most injuries and usually it is rest that did the trick, but they'll try to attribute their recovery to anything but rest.

We devalue the rest cure because we dread it. Most of us would rather be told there is some exercise, some stretching, some piece of gear or, best of all, a pill, that will get us back on the road. The last thing we want to hear is that in order to get back to running we have to stop running.

But if you take an injury to a conventional medical practitioner, that's the first thing you'll be told. "Stay off it for a while." This person might be a medical doctor, very often a general practitioner, and his or her goal is to make sure you don't hurt yourself to the point where you can't run for a very long time, or perhaps the rest of your life. True, hurting yourself to that extent is a dire and unlikely scenario, but from this health practitioner's point of view, there is no reason not to practice the most conservative medicine. To his way of thinking complete rest makes perfect sense. Shutting you down for six to eight weeks means he's stopped the activity that is presumably causing the problem and he is allowing your body to do something it is very good at: heal itself.

It's smart science. It's common sense. It's even cost effective.

But there may be important information this health practitioner doesn't have, especially if the two of you are not well acquainted, and particularly if he or she is not a runner.

RUNNING IS HEALTHY

❶ *Running is mistaken to be the cause of some ailments it not only **does not** cause, but that it may help to prevent. For instance, many people, health practitioners included, think running can diminish joint health and lead to arthritis. Studies show the opposite is true: running does not cause arthritis and can help maintain and improve healthy joints.*

❷ *Running has proven to maintain and improve cardiovascular health.*

❸ *Running helps us live longer.*

❹ *Running improves our mood, and how we feel mentally and emotionally has an effect on how effectively our bodies heal.*

Our strategy regarding rest should be like twin pillars, strong and balanced, supporting our approach to the sport. On the one side, yes, of course, let's build rest into our training programs. Rest leads to better and more enjoyable performances when we are running, and rest also is the best way to avoid injuries in the first place.

If you look at the simple training programs we've designed for the Pasadena Pacers (available at pasadenapacers.org) you'll see that most only call for three days of running per week. The other four days are devoted to cross-training, walking or hiking, and complete rest. This holds true for our pre-conditioning program, where we begin with mostly walking and build to five miles running, to our marathon programs, and includes all our intermediate distance programs in between.

On the other side, I want to honor your desire to run and to that end the purpose for this book is not have us all be "nervous Nellies," and say, "If it doesn't feel quite right, shut it down." My purpose is to keep you running. You'll find many tips and strategies here designed to keep you out on the road through the small bumps, twinges and bruises.

Finally, I'm not talking about a mindset resigned to having a minor, chronic injury and running anyway for an indefinite period of time. It's great to pick a race you want to run in the future, set goals and jump into a training program to help you get there. Ramping up to this level of intensity is fun, we often do it with a group, adding to the enjoyment, and it increases our fitness. It also increases the likelihood of injury.

A big part of my intention is to help you bridge from a point midway through your training program, where an injury requires you to scale back or stop running, to a point later in the program when you can resume at 100 percent without having hurt yourself so badly (or missed so much training) that you have to abandon the program and your goal to run the race.

As you gain more experience and become more adept at listening to your body, you will find that sweet spot where you're not afraid of knocking off for a couple days if something doesn't feel quite right, and at the same time you'll know when to push yourself to do a little more than you ever have before.

Running is
the greatest
metaphor for life,
because you get
out of it what
you put into it.

OPRAH WINFREY

CHAPTER 3

Preventing & Treating Common Injuries

WE ARE WORKING TOWARD a perfect world where it is common for people to take up running, fall in love with the sport and run for years without losing a single day to injury. But we're not there yet, not by a long shot. Most of us are going to suffer some kind of injury at some point in our running careers. For those who are new to running it may happen sooner rather than later. In this chapter you'll find a description of the most common injuries runners have to deal with, and some sound advice on what to do if you start to suffer from these symptoms.

ILLIOTIBIAL BAND SYNDROME (ITBS)

The knee is the most common trouble spot for runners and ITBS, which affects the knee, is the most common running ailment of all. If you have been running for any length of time, you've either had it or know someone who has.

But ITBS doesn't just afflict longtime runners. It afflicts newer runners too, especially those who sign up for the kind of marathon training programs that take you from the couch to the finish line in just five months. It's a story told in my office by countless enthusiastic but heartbroken new runners. ITBS tends to show up late in the training programs of these ambitious newcomers, after the runner has done the first 14- or 16-miler. The onset of ITBS is tricky because while it's triggered by that first long weekend run in the half-marathon range, 14 or 16 miles, it doesn't show up until a few days later. Rather, that long run goes very well, and the runner is exhilarated. "Wow, I just ran 16 miles—I'm more than half way to marathon distance, and I feel great!"

Then Tuesday comes and on a much shorter run, seemingly from out of nowhere—bang!—knee pain. "Why is this happening on a piddly six-miler?" the runner wonders. But the pain is real, the only remedy is rest, and two weekends, or maybe four weekends later, the runner makes her comeback and faces a 20- or 22-miler. But she's lost some of her fitness during her down-time, missed an important long run or two, and she's behind in the program. This run doesn't go so well and, depending on how her knee feels, there is a good chance she's too far behind in the program to be ready for the big race.

It's a common scenario and another case of hard work, great intentions and early success brought down by ITBS.

Before we go further, here's a word of caution. Because ITBS is so typical among runners, it seems every website, every health practitioner and every runner is spouting alleged expertise about the problem. Doubt them all.

There are many reasons for the spread of bad information. One is that rest is a miracle cure. It works almost every time. But whatever a runner is doing (in addition to resting) frequently gets the credit for his or her "cure." Runners are so happy to be back out on the roads, they want to tell everyone about their "cure." Consequently, if a runner is practicing the Old Reliable Milkshake Cure—a chocolate milkshake every evening between 7:30 and 8 p.m.—and after ten milkshakes (and ten days of not running) he is as good as new, guess what all his running buddies, including three or four with sore knees, are going to be hearing about?

Another problem is that although ITBS is by far the most common knee problem, a sore knee doesn't necessarily mean you've got ITBS. You'd be surprised how many runners make that mistake. When you don't have much information, it's easy to leap to the wrong conclusion.

The best approach to understanding ITBS and your own knee pain is to read, listen and pay attention to your body carefully. Since every runner's gait and stride are different, it's impossible to guess what the underlying cause of your particular ITBS is. You will have to learn about the syndrome and measure what you know against your symptoms, and your understanding of your body and your characteristics as a runner.

All right, here we go.

ITBS: HOW IT WORKS

The iliotibial band is the thick tendon arising from the group of hip muscles running along the outside of the thigh from the hip to the tibia, the larger of the two leg bones beneath the knee. The purpose of the IT band is to stabilize the knee and hip and hold the knee in place so it can flex properly.

To understand some of the things that can go wrong, let's look at how your body moves while you're running.

Running is a one-sided activity insofar as only one foot is in contact with the ground at a time. When your foot strikes the ground, you are, in essence, balancing on one leg and the other side of your body is suspended in space. The muscles that hold you in this position are the gluteals, psoas, abs and a small muscle on the side of your hip called the tensor fascia latae. If any of these muscles are weak, your hip will drift too far laterally, or will rotate downward on the side where you're not in contact with the ground, and overstretch the iliotibial band. This isn't usually a problem for shorter-distance runners, but when you are tired, such as near the end of a long run, your muscles fail to hold your form and that's when the trouble begins.

As your knee passes back and forth beneath the overstretched IT band, the bony prominence plucks it repeatedly, like a finger playing a stringed instrument, and it creates pain and inflammation (not music) at the attachments.

ITBS: PROBLEMS & SYMPTOMS

The problem of ITBS is friction. It's tendon rubbing on bone. When the IT band becomes too short and tense, when it is pulled in the wrong direction or manner, it rubs on the side of the knee and becomes inflamed just above the spot where it joins the knee. This hurts. It feels like a burning and/or an aching on the outside of the knee, even though it isn't the knee itself that is in pain, but the muscles connecting to it.

If you think of your knee as a clock facing outward, the pain usually begins at about 10 o'clock—in other words, near the top of the knee and on the outside. It hurts to run at first, and later it can hurt to put weight on the knee. Sometimes pain extends upward above the knee along the outside of the thigh, and it intensifies.

The pain usually begins a few days to a week after a long run. Most runners will be baffled as to why they had no trouble on Saturday's 16-miler, but find themselves in pain on Tuesday evening when they are only going four miles. The injury typically occurs during a long run but isn't severe enough to cause pain during normal activity afterward, and doesn't show itself until the next run.

ITBS: CAUSES

ITBS has two main causes and several others that are less frequently seen but just as troublesome when they appear. The first main cause is ***over-pronating***. When you over-pronate, your leg twists very slightly toward a midline that you can envision running forward directly beneath the center of your body. When you over-pronate, your right knee twists slightly counter-clockwise and your left knee twists clock-wise, with each step. Over-pronating puts too much pressure on the inside of each foot. You'll see the wear showing unevenly on the inner portions of your shoes.

If you imagine over-pronating, with your knee twisting inward, you can almost feel a pull on the outside of your thigh where the muscles join the knee. To understand this better, stand up and roll your feet in and out while holding your hand on the outside of the thigh. That's the sensation of your iliotibial band being pulled and most likely stretching over the bony end of your femur where it joins your knee. The result is friction, irritation, inflammation, soreness and pain.

ITBS very often begins near the end of an unusually long run, or at some other point when you are piling on the mileage. A typical scenario is that your form breaks down, your posture and your gait are affected, and you wind up putting strain on your illiotibial band.

The second cause of ITBS is ***weak core and hip muscles***. Your iliopsoas muscles wrap around from your back to the front of your body and slide down the face of your lower abdomen, attaching to the inside of the thigh. They are crucial posture muscles, important not only for running, but simply standing and walking. If they are weak, your forward movement will be compromised and there will be too much left-right pelvic sway in your gait. The muscles on the outside of your hips, including your iliotibial band, will become overloaded, creating excess tension at the attachment point. The same chain reaction as with over-pronating will occur: friction, irritation, inflammation, soreness and pain.

A third cause of ITBS is ***running on a crowned surface***. Typically, we run on asphalt roads in residential neighborhoods. The closer you run to the center of the road, the more level the surface will be. If you run on the outside of the road, close to the gutter, you may find yourself on a slanted surface on which one leg is extending down a couple inches below the other in order to reach the road. Avoid these surfaces because they are damaging to your legs and back; instead find safe, level surfaces on which to run. *(See more on running safety in chapter 4.)*

ILLIOTIBIAL BAND SYNDROME (ITBS)

When the IT band becomes too short and tense, when it is pulled in the wrong direction or manner, it rubs on the side of the knee and becomes inflamed just above the spot where it joins the knee.

Symptoms

A burning and/or an aching on the outside of the knee, even though it isn't the knee itself that is in pain, but the muscles connecting to it.

Causes

- Over-pronating
- Weak core and hip muscles
- Uneven running surface
- Weak gluteal muscles
- Short leg
- Severe ankle sprain

Treatment & Solutions

- Scale back on mileage. Increase more slowly
- New and/or better shoes
- Insoles, arch supports or orthotics
- Strengthen your core through cross-training
- Strengthen weak hip muscles
- Strengthen weak ankles
- Stretching and self-massage
- Use a foam roller to stretch the outside of the thigh
- Ice the sore area after running
- Use a heel lift to compensate for one leg that is shorter

If you have **weak gluteal muscles** your leg may sway during the swing phase of your gait, resulting in your foot being out of alignment when you land. If the foot crosses the midline prior to the strike phase, you will over-supinate, meaning land with too much pressure on the outside of your foot. This will also bring your iliotibial band out of alignment and start the muscle-on-bone sequence. *(See the Side Plank exercise on page 123 to strengthen gluteal muscles.)*

Many people have **one leg shorter than the other**; it's a common occurrence and it usually doesn't lead to problems. However, when one leg is nine centimeters shorter (about one-third of an inch), problems are likely to occur. The illiotibial band on the short leg may become sore because it's being unnaturally stretched laterally. *(See Short-Leg Syndrome on page 62.)*

A **severely sprained ankle**, even when thought to have completely healed months or years in the past, can cause poor control of the foot and misaligned biomechanics. Sensors in the tendons relay important information to the brain regarding the foot's position in space, and often after a bad ankle sprain these sensors never fully heal. The result is poor alignment at the foot strike.

ITBS: TREATMENTS AND SOLUTIONS

Ice the sore area

For all the problems associated with the IT band, there is one advantage in treating it. Since it's close to the surface it is easy to treat with ice. The ice has a more direct and therefore greater effect. Ten minutes applying ice is usually enough to cool it and calm the inflammation.

I like to use a solid block of ice so I can massage the IT band while cooling it; with a solid block in nearly direct contact you'll probably only need four to seven minutes of application and massage.

Fill a Styrofoam or paper cup with water and freeze it, then peel away half an inch from the top portion of the cup and you'll have a perfectly sized and shaped piece of ice to work with. Use a thin towel when it begins to drip, then put it back in the freezer until next time.

Take NSAIDs

Over the counter, non-steroidal, anti-inflammatory drugs (brand names like Advil, Ibuprofen, and Aleve) really work. They can be very helpful with the initial inflammatory phase of ITBS, so go ahead and use them.

It's fine to have them as a regular item in your runner's equipment bag. I don't have a quarrel with middle-aged runners who take one or two before heading out on a particularly long or arduous run, or a race.

What NSAIDs are not, and you should not let them become, is a substitute for discovering and treating the cause of some pain that is chronic or acute. Pain is an early warning sign that something is wrong, and taking a pill and ignoring it is never a good idea.

Stretching and self-massage

If you have ITBS, in addition to the muscles rubbing on bone, the muscles may have become shorter and tighter than normal. Stretching the iliotibial band is not as easy as stretching a large, available muscle like a calf or a hamstring. In fact, the ITB is a tough piece of anatomy that is anything but stretchy. It is a ligament and like all ligaments it's not intended to stretch very much. (If they did, they would not provide good joint stability, which is their job.)

This doesn't mean you shouldn't do your best to stretch it out. But don't be frustrated if you don't feel that obvious pull on the muscle on the outside of your leg. Because of the physiology, it won't be that no-doubt-about-it tug you get in your hamstrings when you bend over to touch your toes. Still, you can lengthen and relax your ITB with a number of stretches. *(See ITB exercises on page 121-124.)*

Many runners report feeling better when they use a foam roller. Add it to your repertoire of treatments and you will increase your chances of experiencing relief. There is a great line of self-massage tools called "The Stick." They come in a variety of shapes and sizes but essentially they are rolling pins to help you loosen, lengthen and restore tight or pulled muscles. Using a roller on the outside of your thigh will relax your iliotibial band and speed healing.

Adjust mileage and intensity

Check to see if you are over-pronating due to poor biomechanics caused by fatigue. At the end of a long run, have someone make a video of you running half a block or so. Ask someone knowledgeable about proper form to look at the video and evaluate your gait. Your local independent running store is your most likely source for someone who can spot proper biomechanics. Schools, colleges and running clubs are other possibilities.

If fatigue is causing you to lapse into improper form, scale back on your mileage and increase more slowly. For most runners, increasing by approximately 10% per week is reasonable but this may not apply to every runner and every circumstance. Training programs can appear one way on paper or the computer screen but be very different on the roads.

Your natural ability as a runner, your general level of fitness and your age will determine how quickly you can increase your mileage, much more so than numbers on a chart in a training plan.

Be careful of the tendency to "adjust" the numbers for the sake of keeping up. If you get sick in Week #4 and miss a week of training, don't expect to take on the Week #6 workouts as if you had never been away.

Also pay attention to the length of each workout. There is a big difference between a 12-mile week made up of three 4-mile runs, versus a 12-mile week consisting of one 3-mile run and a Saturday 9-miler. In general, the 10% per week guideline should apply to the long run as well the weekly total.

A final concern is the intensity of your workouts. Intensity means speed. It's a good idea, especially if you are new to running, to work out well below your ability level. If you run for 10 miles at a speed that prevents you from carrying on a conversation except in gasps, you are probably loading on too much speed. Likewise, sprinting the last quarter mile is unwise. Be especially careful near the ends of your runs because this is when you are most fatigued and, hence, your form is at its weakest. When your gait is at its most misaligned is when you are putting maximum stress on your joints, tendons and muscles. This is when injuries are most likely to occur, and when they occur most quickly.

Try different shoes or arch supports
Check to see if you are over-pronating due to a natural inconsistency in your biomechanics. Take an old pair of shoes into your independent running store. Someone there will check the wear patterns and quickly determine whether or not you regularly over-pronate. If you do, a different or better pair of shoes may correct the problem. An off-the-shelf arch support might also provide a solution. Either one can provide a cushion that evens out your inward stride.

Use off-the-shelf or custom orthotics
An orthotic can provide enough support to restore balance to your stride and take the strain off your iliotibial band. I advise trying an off-the-shelf insole or orthotic before choosing a custom-designed orthotic because they often provide sufficient correction but cost only $20 to $50, versus ten times that amount for orthotics fitted in a doctor's or podiatrist's office. Off-the-shelf orthotics are molded cushions that fit into the bottom of your shoe like an insole and improve alignment as your feet strike the ground.

Strengthen core muscles
In recent years, the growth of Pilates has raised awareness of the importance of

strong core muscles. A yoga studio is also a good place to work on abdominals and core strength. Bicycling is another great choice. When your feet are clipped onto bicycle pedals, each up stroke precisely strengthens the psoas muscles that help support and stabilize the iliotibial band. Seated leg raises and lateral leg raises strengthen hip muscles and iliopsoas muscles, also important for ITB support. *(See Leg Raise exercise on page 135.)* Rollerblading is another great cross-training exercise for ITB support.

Strengthen hip muscles

Stand on your left leg and raise your right knee until your foot is even with your left knee. Take a moment to feel stable and then lower your right hip. If this exercise is difficult for you, if you can't do 20 repeats, your hip muscles may need strengthening. Another check is to lie down, raise one leg and attempt to press it outward against resistance provided by a friend. If you have trouble applying a good amount of pressure, hip strengtheners are for you. *(See exercises beginning on page 143.)*

Strengthen ankle tendons

If you can predict a weather change by an ache in one of your ankles, and if you have experience on the football field or the basketball, volleyball or tennis court, you're probably carrying the effects of a badly sprained ankle. This means the tendons around your ankle are not fully functioning and it is very likely that with time and increased mileage, the inability of your ankles to maintain proper foot, knee and leg alignment will create trouble in your calves, knees and iliotibial band.

Sprained ankles are not memorable. Many don't require an x-ray. They heal within a few days or a couple weeks at most, and it seems as if there are no long-term consequences. But a serious sprained ankle can leave your ligaments compromised, and years later when you begin running, your gait is slightly off.

Here is an exercise that will help you assess and improve the strength of your ankles:

Stand on a stair with your ankles and heels hanging off the edge. Now try raising yourself with one foot. If it's too difficult start with both feet and keep at it until you can do 15 repeats with one foot. Also, lying down try to move a heavy piece of furniture first to the left and then to the right with the same ankle. These exercises will strengthen your tendons and help stabilize your biomechanics.

Correct pelvic alignment

Sometimes you can feel an imbalance in your pelvis. It feels like one side of

Heavy Usage: Why Runners Court the Risk of Injury

A sedentary person can take as few as 1,000 steps (and cover less than a mile) per day. On a typical Saturday, a Pasadena Pacer takes 7,000 steps (approximately five miles) before breakfast. In the thick of marathon training, that number could easily shoot up to 20,000 to 30,000.

To put it very simply, runners take more steps and use their legs and feet more than other people. What's more, a running step takes more of a toll on the hips, legs, knees, ankles and feet than a normal step because it brings greater impact. While our exercise brings great benefits to our bodies, minds and spirits, there is also a cost, namely, heavier usage of our bodies.

It doesn't cost money to go out for a run, but there is a price we should pay on a daily basis and that is greater vigilance over our health. You are right to be reading this book and you do well when you apply what you find here. The first part of being vigilant is paying attention to your body. The second is responding when you notice a symptom that could be telling you something.

The 15 minutes of icing while you read or watch TV, the extra five minutes of stretching, the $100 massage, the yoga class or pool workout could save you weeks lost to injury.

your pelvic area is more forward than the other. It's a common occurrence that won't affect most people, but it can restrict the backward leg swing when you run and that will put undo stress on the knee. If you have this out-of-alignment sensation, the best thing to do is get an adjustment from a chiropractor, and do it before you experience pain in your knees or legs.

Cross-train

Cross-training on a bike, rollerblading, yoga, swimming or strength training in a gym almost completely eliminates the risk of having ITBS. Start your cross-training early and you will complete your race training program with less risk of IT band trouble.

Run on a flat surface

Many roads are crowned, in other words, higher in the middle and lower on the sides. They can be so crowned, in fact, that when you run on the left side of the road, facing traffic, your right foot is closer to the pavement by as much as two or three inches. Running in this position is like having your right leg that much shorter than your left, and it will definitely throw your gait out of alignment.

If you are having ITB pain and you suspect an uneven surface could be the culprit, then find a track, a treadmill or a trail—some surface you are certain is flat—and run on it as an experiment to see if your pain abates.

Seek professional therapy

When nothing else is working, it is time for a trip to a health practitioner who specializes in working with athletes, especially runners. The person you seek out might be a physical therapist, chiropractor, trainer, massage therapist or medical doctor.

If you have persistent knee pain a good physical therapist, or any of these other practitioners, should be able to observe your biomechanics and diagnose your problem.

I think of all forms of treatment by a practitioner as tactics you don't want to resort to until you've run out of other alternatives because they are expensive and don't always treat the underlying cause.

Once you've decided to see a professional therapist, make sure you find one who has plenty of experience with runners. The best-case scenario is to find a health practitioner who is a runner himself or herself.

◆ ◆ ◆

THE KNEE

Knee problems are among the most common running injuries. Maintaining clean, abundant, healthy cartilage is the best thing we can do to keep our knees in good shape. The two best ways to take care of your cartilage are: make sure you are running in alignment, and with sufficiently cushioned shoes. This means replacing your shoes when they become worn or feel like they've gotten hard and lost their spring, their pizzazz.

Danger signs indicating serious knee problems include locking, where you can't fully straighten your knee, and a clicking sound that could indicate an internal joint problem. Swelling in the back of the knee is also a red flag, and so is pain along the joint line.

However, most knee problems runners face occur slowly, over time, and are chronic rather than acute.

ARTHRITIS IN THE KNEE

First, despite occasional claims to the contrary, running does not cause arthritis. In fact, some studies indicate that exercise, including running, helps promote and prolong the health and longevity of cartilage. Here is a link to an article in *Time* magazine about an important long-term study done at Stanford University that helps set the record straight—http://www.time.com/time/health/article/0,8599,1948208,00.html.

Knee cartilage is the elastic connective tissue in the joint that allows the hinge to swing freely with a minimum of friction. Cartilage is like the body's Teflon. Things don't adhere to it.

Osteoarthritis occurs when the knee cartilage begins to wear away and the bones—the femur and the tibia—get too close. At first this creates inflammation and causes pain. Eventually, the joint can wear down and the bones get so close they are rubbing. Osteoarthritis is the most common form of knee arthritis and the type most likely to affect runners. It occurs due to accumulated wear and tear. Its onset is usually gradual and accumulative.

Two other kinds of arthritis that can affect the knee are rheumatoid arthritis, an inflammatory arthritis that can occur suddenly and often affects both knees, and post-traumatic arthritis, which is due to a knee injury and can occur years after the trauma.

BURSITIS

Bursitis is inflammation of a bursa, a small sac filled with fluid—think mini water balloons—that reduces friction and cushions pressure points between

continued on page 144

ARTHRITIS IN THE KNEE

Osteoarthritis occurs when the knee cartilage begins to wear away and the bones—the femur and the tibia—get too close. At first this creates inflammation and causes pain. Eventually, the joint can wear down and the bones get so close they are rubbing. Osteoarthritis is the most common form of knee arthritis and the type most likely to affect runners.

Symptoms

- Pain present first thing in the morning
- Pain consistently present after exertion
- Pain present in cold, damp weather
- Stiff, swollen knee joint, difficult to straighten or bend
- Pain increase after running

Causes

- An erosion of the knee cartilage between the femur and tibia

Treatment & Solutions

- Scale back on mileage. Increase more slowly
- An x-ray will tell how much cartilage loss you've suffered
- Weight loss, if appropriate (the less weight the legs must support, the less stress there is on the knee joint)
- Strengthen the muscles around the knee to minimize impact on the joint
- Stretch the muscles around the joint
- Pain relievers such as NSAIDs
- Run on trails and/or other soft surfaces

BURSITIS

Bursitis is inflammation of a bursa, a small sac filled with fluid—think mini water balloons—that reduces friction and cushions pressure points between muscles and/or tendons and bone.

Symptoms

- Pain or tenderness where the knee meets the quadriceps
- Hurts to swing the knee joint and/or put weight on it
- Area can feel swollen, even squishy
- Sometimes the area feels warm to the touch from the inflammation

Causes

- Most likely cause for runners is excess training on hills
- A secondary cause is poor form, particularly one foot crossing the mid-line
- Too many exercises that put too much stress on joints, such as high-intensity lunges or squats, done while supporting a maximum amount of weights

Treatment & Solutions

- Rest
- Ice
- Reduce hill running
- Quality, properly fitted shoes

PATELLAR TRACKING PROBLEMS

The patella is your kneecap and if it shifts or tilts incorrectly when you bend or straighten your knee it will track crooked in its groove, creating a painful experience.

Symptoms

- Pain in the knee
- Pain at the medial (central portion) knee, just below the kneecap
- Pain at the medial or just to the inside of the patellar tendon

Causes

- Imperfectly formed patella. There are several different architectural styles of kneecaps, and some are more prone to tracking and dislocation
- Weak medial quadriceps muscles
- Tight tendons or muscles in the legs, feet or hips, such as the IT band
- A blow to the kneecap (old football or soccer injuries)
- Pronating or supinating, causing misalignment

Treatment & Solutions

- Strengthening exercises for your medial quadriceps
- Ice
- Stretch before and after running (particularly thigh muscles, IT band, hamstrings and Achilles tendon)
- Correct gait so the knee will track properly (over-pronating can be corrected with arch supports, orthotics or a more supportive running shoe)

muscles and/or tendons and bone.

There are several bursae within the knee. The one most likely to be affected by running is at the top of the kneecap close to the quadriceps.

PATELLAR TRACKING PROBLEMS

The patella is your kneecap and if it shifts or tilts incorrectly when you bend or straighten your knee it will track crooked in its groove, creating a painful experience.

Beneath your kneecap there is a groove and the underside of your kneecap fits neatly into this groove. In some people—and this can easily be determined by a particular type of x-ray—the groove is too shallow. Rather than fitting securely into the groove, because of the shallowness of the groove, the connection is naturally loose.

If you experience habitual soreness beneath or around your kneecap, it is worth your while to have a "sunrise x-ray" taken of your knee.

◆ ◆ ◆

LEG INJURIES

"SHIN SPLINTS"

"Shin splints" over the years has become a catch-all term for pain in the muscles or tendons running along the front of the tibia—the shin. The pain usually runs down the bottom third of the tibia. Vertical pain usually means the injury is occurring in the muscles and/or tendons. Pain that runs across the leg below the knee might indicate a stress fracture.

Usually with shin splints, you feel the pain as soon as you begin running but it often lessens as the run progresses. Then it feels worse a day or two later as you head out for your next run. In essence, it's not good that the pain abates so you can finish your run, because that cycle enables you to make the injury worse.

Ignoring the pain of shin splints is a particularly bad idea because they can worsen and become stress fractures, which is a much more serious injury.

STRESS FRACTURES IN THE LOWER LEG

Stress fractures are tiny cracks in the bone caused over time by a continued, repetitive force that is more taxing than the bone can withstand. Running is a classic example. Stress fractures usually require an MRI to diagnose and can take weeks to heal. Avoid them by paying careful attention to pain in the lower leg that radiates laterally.

SHIN SPLINTS

Over the years "shin splints" has become a catch-all term for pain in the muscles or tendons running along the front of the tibia—the shin. The pain usually runs down the bottom third of the tibia. Vertical pain usually means the injury is occurring in the muscles and/or tendons. Pain that runs across the leg below the knee might indicate a stress fracture.

Symptoms

- Tenderness, soreness or pain in the lower leg
- Occasionally, swelling in the affected area
- Often lumps are present in the shin muscles (you can feel them when you run your fingers along the inside of the shin)

Causes

- Tight foot muscles
- High arches
- Worn-out shoes
- Running on slanted or tilted surfaces

Treatment & Solutions

- Rest
- Ice
- Quality running shoes properly fitted for your particular stride
- Stretch before and after running
- Compression sleeves (sometimes called "compression socks" or "'calf sleeves") can provide support to the calf muscles while reducing stress on the shin
- Arch supports or orthotics can help cushion your leg and disperse the stress
- Strengthen the tendons that support the arch of the foot
- Taping
- Self-massage along the shin muscle, but avoid putting pressure on the bone

RISK FACTORS
STRESS FRACTURES

- *Flat feet*

- *High, rigid arches*

- *Osteoporosis*

- *Participating in other high-impact sports (basketball, tennis, etc.)*

- *A sudden shift from a sedentary lifestyle to high activity*

If you suspect you have a stress fracture, stop running right away, even if you are in the middle of a workout. Since stress fractures develop over time, rest, ice, adding mileage slowly or reducing mileage when necessary can prevent them from occurring in the first place.

◆ ◆ ◆

ANKLE INJURIES

When the Divine Design team was putting together the human body they had to strike a balance between strength and flexibility with each structural system. For muscles, they favored flexibility, for bones, strength. With ligaments, the fibrous tissue that connects bones to one another, they had to walk a middle path. The result is that while ligaments are elastic enough to stretch and tough enough to hold bones together, they are neither flexible enough to stretch and return unhurt when they are pulled, nor strong enough to hold their position when they're strained.

The classic example of this kind of ligament damage is the sprained ankle. If you run on smooth surfaces you aren't at great risk for an ankle sprain, but most of us didn't start fresh as runners. We came to running with the usual team sports of youth in our backgrounds—baseball, volleyball, soccer, tennis, football, basketball, softball, etc. One of the most common injuries in each of these sports is a sprained ankle.

When you twist, turn or roll your ankle beyond its normal range of motion, you pull the ligaments further than they are meant to go, and they get stretched or torn. When they heal they may lose some of their strength and

STRESS FRACTURES

Stress fractures are tiny cracks in the bone caused over time by a continued, repetitive force that is more taxing than the bone can withstand. Diagnosing stress fractures requires special imaging.

Symptoms

- Pain in the leg running laterally (across rather than up and down)
- Pain coming early in the run that is significant, possibly causing you to end the workout
- There's no trauma associated with the pain, ruling out the possibility of a bruise
- The pain is deep and serious, leaving the leg sensitive to the touch
- Pushing on the affected spot is significantly painful
- The pain is too intense for you to hop on the affected leg

Causes

- Pounding and stress on the bones—running is definitely a culprit
- Tugging/pulling at tendons and muscles connected to the leg bones
- Fatigue that causes muscles to break down and diminishes their ability to absorb shock and stress
- Excessively rapid increase in training that leads to or exacerbates conditions described above
- Improper footwear that fails to properly cushion legs

Treatments & Solutions

- Bone pain, especially if it radiates laterally, means **stop running immediately**
- Rest
- Ice
- Strengthening the muscles and tendons connected to and supporting the ankle and the leg, particularly the calf muscles
- May take six to eight weeks to heal

flexibility and other attributes as well.

Having had a serious ankle sprain is the greatest predictor that you could turn your ankle again. If you know you've had one, take special care to run on smooth surfaces. Every running course has at least a couple spots, even if they are only a few steps, where you have to run from curb to street, over grass or a rutted area—be especially cautious as you navigate over these spots.

SPRAINED ANKLES AND "PROPRIOCEPTION" PROBLEMS

There are a number of stretch receptor sites in ankle ligaments including the one that supports the outside and back of the ankle and is so frequently damaged in an ankle sprain.

The stretch receptor sites there give information to your brain about your body's position in space. Your brain interpolates that data and uses it to tense up certain muscles that hold you upright. People with severe sprains have destroyed some of those sites and their sense of position in space is lessened. You've lost some of your sense of balance. Obviously, as runners we want to be as sure-footed as possible. Uncertain footing makes reccurring ankle sprains more likely, which is a bad thing especially if you've suffered a serious sprain in the past. Badly sprained ligaments tend not to heal 100% and that makes them easier to turn or twist, and the sprain happens again.

Weakened proprioception can lead to gait problems, and it makes you more susceptible to other lower leg injuries as well.

A quick preliminary test to check how well your proprioception systems are working is to stand on one leg and close your eyes. You should be able to maintain your balance for 10 seconds.

ACHILLES TENDINITIS

Named after the Greek warrior, Achilles, the large tendon at the back and bottom of the leg connects the calf muscle to the heel and when it becomes inflamed spells real trouble for runners.

Putting a large amount of stress on your Achilles too quickly or too frequently creates tiny tears in the tendon and leads to inflammation.

It's important that your Achilles can stretch sufficiently as you push off to avoid overstressing the tendon.

There is also a bursa in the area that could be the cause of pain or soreness. You can test for bursitis in the heel area by squeezing the back of your ankle where the Achilles attaches to the heel. But don't squeeze the tendon itself, rather

SPRAINED ANKLES AND "PROPRIOCEPTION" PROBLEMS

There are a number of stretch receptor sites in ankle ligaments including the one that supports the outside and back of the ankle and is so frequently damaged in an ankle sprain.

Symptoms

- Occasional sense of unsteady footing due to loss of balance
- Repeat sprains from rolling the foot unnaturally to the left or right

Causes

- Damaged receptor sites in lower legs, usually due to sprains or strains

Treatments & Solutions

- Strengthening muscles around the ankle

squeeze a half inch in front of the tendon, toward the center of your foot. If this is the tender spot, as opposed to the tendon at the far back, then it's probably an inflamed bursa.

If so, a shoe with a heel cup that is too tight or with ill-fitting padding against the heel may be to blame. Ice and a better pair of shoes should resolve the problem.

Is your Achilles flexible enough? In order to properly execute the end of your push-off phase, you have to be able to flex your heel 12-15 degrees. You can test your flexing ability sitting down by extending your leg and holding the bottom of your foot perpendicular to your leg. Now flex the top of your foot toward your knee. If you can stretch your toe all the way back until it touches your shin— highly unlikely—it would cover 90 degrees. For it to travel 15 degrees you have to move it 1/6th that distance. See if you can. If you cannot, work on Achilles stretches for a couple weeks and try again. *(See pages 117-120.)*

◆ ◆ ◆

FOOT INJURIES

Ah, the humble foot. Not given its due until something goes wrong.

John Wooden, arguably the greatest coach in the history of college athletics, knew better. He began the first practice of every basketball season with a lesson on how to properly put on socks and lace up sneakers.

Basketball great Michael Jordan, legendary for his unwillingness to leave the court, missed games on more than one occasion because of an infected foot. A simple tear in the skin once led to an infection that landed Air Jordan in the hospital on IV antibiotics.

Nowhere in the human body is there so much engineering packed into such a small space as in the foot—26 bones, 33 joints and more than 100 ligaments.

If your stride is approximately three feet in length, you can count on each foot landing on the pavement more than 750 times per mile. The force of impact on your feet depends in part on your weight.

With all our feet have to endure, and with so many points of potential complication, it behooves us to pay attention to our feet, take common-sense precautions and don't neglect them when they need special care. When ignored, foot injuries tend to worsen and lead to complications.

PLANTAR FASCIITIS

Your plantar fascia is the tough membrane just beneath the surface of your skin that runs the length of the bottom of your foot. It spans your arch and connects

ACHILLES TENDINITIS

The large tendon at the back and bottom of the leg connects the calf muscle to the heel. Putting a large amount of stress on your Achilles too quickly or too frequently creates tiny tears in the tendon and leads to inflammation.

Symptoms

- A dull ache or pain in the tendon running down into your heel when pushing off as you begin walking, the sensitivity increasing in intensity as you run.
- Tenderness to the touch

Causes

- Overuse in various forms
- If your calf muscles are too weak or inflexible, the Achilles tendon may be overloaded with stress as you run
- If you are new to running or begin a more ambitious training program, too many miles added on too quickly could overstress your Achilles
- Running on hills or in sand or other soft surfaces, including grass, tends to overload the Achilles tendon and can cause inflammation

Treatment & Solutions

- Rest
- Ice
- Compression wraps or elastic bandages can help ease the swelling
- An orthotic device or a heel lift can relieve strain on the over-stretched tendon (raising the heel will reduce the angle your tendon has to achieve in order to create push-off; if you use a heel lift, make sure you use one on each side and that they match)
- A night splint will help keep the tendons stretched during the night
- Stretching the tendon and other heel muscles
- NSAIDs such as aspirin, acetaminophen and ibuprofen (be careful about using these medicines continuously for more than one week because many of them carry serious side effects)

your toes to your heel.

The plantar fascia is unique because it is the only ligament in your body that bears the full brunt of your weight and is in direct contact with the earth. Other muscles help absorb the force of your weight against the ground, but your plantar fascia is the only one that takes on all your weight while being pushed straight into the ground. If it becomes inflamed it will be sensitive to pressure and that will certainly mean pain when you try to run. It's very possible it will hurt to walk or even stand.

The most dramatic feature of plantar fasciitis is the "first step sign." When you take your first step in the morning the arch is exquisitely painful. This can also happen if you've been sitting for a long time. No one knows definitively why this occurs but one belief is that running or walking can cause micro-tears in the fascia. Overnight, these very small tears heal, but are ruptured again with the first steps in the morning.

Every runner's fear regarding this injury is that it will take a long time to fully recover from it. Sometimes plantar fasciitis does become a nagging, recurring injury. Therefore, the best approach is to take the first signs seriously and begin treatment right away.

Collapsing arches, which are a normal part of the aging process, can also lead to plantar fasciitis. Over time, our feet flatten out, our shoe sizes get larger and it can lead to stretching of the ligaments on the bottom of the foot.

PLANTAR FASCIA STRETCH

For 20 seconds every hour. Reach your big toe toward your knee and hold for a few seconds, then reach it down as if trying to touch your heel.

This technique will be most effective if you do it many times during the day.

Wearing a night splint can keep your plantar fascia and Achilles elongated while you sleep. Based on the presumption that small tears in the fascia heal improperly while your foot is in a relaxed position overnight, only to tear again as soon as you flex and put weight on your foot in the morning, a night splint is a device that is designed to keep your foot stretched overnight.

They come in various configurations but most involve a wrap that extends

PLANTAR FASCIITIS

Other muscles help absorb the force of your weight against the ground, but your plantar fascia is the only one that takes on all your weight while being pushed straight into the ground. When inflamed it will be sensitive to pressure and that will certainly mean pain when you try to run.

Symptoms

- May develop gradually with onset in the form of soreness along the arch of the foot
- Worst pain comes with the first step in the morning or after prolonged periods of sitting or lying down, such as a long car ride
- Usually affects one foot although it can affect both feet simultaneously
- Pain feels sharp, in the arch and/or heel

Causes

- Over-pronation
- Sudden increase in distance or speed
- Fascia is too short or stretched too taut
- Tight Achilles tendon or calf muscles can overstress the plantar fascia
- Collapsing arch

Treatment & Solutions

- Stretch the muscles in the bottom of your foot throughout the day using the stretch technique described on page 52
- Stretching exercises for the plantar fascia and Achilles on pages 117-120
- Wearing a night splint can keep your plantar fascia and Achilles elongated while you sleep
- Orthotics, either off-the-shelf or custom-fitted, can distribute the pressure more evenly to all parts of the foot
- Stretching and/or strengthening the muscles in the lower leg can also help absorb the pressure of impact
- NSAIDs may help relieve pain but will not address underlying causes

around the foot and up around the ankle. Some have a strap that extends from the top of your foot to your ankle as a way to keep the foot from straightening too much. If you work at a desk you can wear it there during the day as well. Choose a night splint with a hard shell; they are far more effective.

METATARSALGIA (AND FRACTURE OF THE 5TH METATARSAL BONE)

If you press into the bottom of your foot just beneath the toes, about even with the ball of your foot, you will feel five small bones, one connecting each toe to the rest of the foot. These are the metatarsal bones. To the touch, the rounded head of each metatarsal feels like a piece of pea gravel.

Metatarsalgia is inflammation in and around these small bones that causes pain in the ball of your foot. If you feel pain and soreness in this area, and one or more of your metatarsals are too sore to press, stop running. There is the possibility of a stress fracture. If you run on a stress fracture the bone could shatter.

Pay particular attention to the fifth metatarsal, beneath your smallest toe near the outside of your foot, because this is where a stress fracture is most likely to occur.

Stress fractures are hard to diagnose but often you won't need to. It will simply heal over time, perhaps as long as ten weeks. These are weight-bearing bones and therefore slower to heal. If you do not have a stress fracture, metatarsalgia is not a serious problem and should resolve itself within a couple weeks.

If the soreness is away from the metatarsal bone and lower on your foot, closer to your heel, you have tendonitis, not metatarsalgia.

STRESS FRACTURES IN THE FOOT

In a conventional fracture, there is a break that shows on the outside of the bone. But think of the bone as a cylinder and imagine a break that begins on the inside and does not penetrate all the way through so that it shows on the outside. This is a stress fracture. In general, it is difficult to diagnose a stress fracture with an x-ray; the best way to detect them is with an MRI.

SESAMOIDITIS

Sesamoid bones are shaped like sesame seeds and thus, their name. They are found in several locations in the body where a tendon passes over a joint, such as the hand, knee and foot. There are two sesamoid bones around the big toe joint under the ball of your foot. Like kneecaps, which are also sesamoid bones, they act as force multipliers.

Roll your thumb back and forth over this area and you can feel the sesamoid

METATARSALGIA

There are five metatarsal bones, one connecting each toe to your foot. Metatarsalgia is inflammation in and around these small bones that causes pain in the ball of your foot.

Symptoms

- Pain in the ball of your foot (may be aching, burning or sharp)
- Running makes the pain worse
- Feels like you are running or walking with a pebble in your shoe

Causes

- Beware the possibility of stress fractures, which can cause these symptoms (see stress fractures, page 54)
- Landing on an object, such as a sharp rock, during a run
- Increasing speed and/or adding distance too quickly
- Too much hill running (since it adds pressure to the front of the foot)
- Shoes that fit poorly or have inadequate padding
- Running on hard surfaces with insufficient cushioning from footwear can damage your feet (with due respect for the latest running trends, beware of running barefoot or with the new ultra-thin shoes that have "fingers" for your toes similar to those of a glove)

Treatment & Solutions

- Rest (swimming and cycling are the go-to workouts of choice when you have a leg or foot injury)
- Ice
- Better shoes (more padding on the soles may help)
- Insoles can add more shock-absorbing padding (the main thing your injured foot needs is protection)
- Teardrop-shaped metatarsal pads carefully positioned in the arch can relieve pressure on the metatarsal heads
- Resume training slowly
- If you have a more serious stress fracture (one that prohibits you from walking) an MRI may be warranted and you should see an orthopedic physician

bone shifting just as your kneecap does. These small sesamoid bones are situated on the bottom of the foot where the big toe joins in. They are subject to becoming inflamed or even fractured. When they do, they'll become sore and painful during the push-off phase of your gait.

BLISTERS

Blisters are caused by friction when something, usually your shoe, rubs against your skin. The first layer of skin is rubbed so raw that it begins to die and your body causes fluid to build up beneath to protect the tender skin below.

Since each foot strikes the ground somewhere between 500 and 1,000 times per mile, if something comes out of alignment and begins to rub during a run, you can develop a blister in a matter of minutes.

They usually begin with a "hot spot," a place where you can feel heat focused in a small area. If you catch the blister during this phase, before the skin begins to separate and fluid builds up, you can prevent it from developing into a full-blown blister. Unfortunately, most runners are like kids on the playground who don't want to stop having fun even to go to the bathroom. But if you are savvy enough to detect a hot spot and can make yourself do the right thing, stop and treat yourself right away. Blister first-aid materials, such as adhesive bandages, moleskin, tape or a small tube of petroleum jelly, weigh almost nothing, and since they can mean the difference between completing a run and taking a long, painful walk home, I carry a small supply in my shorts pockets or fuel belt.

The first remedy is to stop the rubbing. Ironically, shoes that are either too big or too tight can create rubbing. If your shoes are too large, your feet can slip upon impact, creating rubbing. More likely for runners is finding ourselves in shoes that are too small. With each step in a tight shoe, the foot wears against the inside of the shoe.

Runners are creatures of habit and we get used to wearing the same size shoe. But over time our feet change, usually getting bigger, and we don't notice our shoes becoming tighter. If you are over 40, your arches have probably flattened somewhat, making your feet longer. If you've gone through a pregnancy, you know how much your feet can expand.

I've seen many runners so desensitized to the fit of their shoes that they have worn an indentation in the tip from impact with their big toe. I call this bump a "wear bulb."

SESAMOIDITIS

Small sesamoid bones are situated on the bottom of the foot where the big toe joins in. They are subject to becoming inflamed or even fractured. When they do, they'll become sore and painful during the push-off phase of your gait.

Symptoms

- Pain and soreness on the very bottom of the ball of your foot
- The feeling of having a rock in your shoe

Causes

- High arches
- Over-pronation
- Any gait flaw that causes poor shock absorption
- Shoes with insufficient cushioning
- Tight calf muscles
- Bunions, which shift more pressure to the sesamoid bones

Treatment & Solutions

- Make sure the cushioning in your shoes is not overly worn
- Change to shoes with softer, more cushioned insoles
- Add an insole that provides additional cushioning
- Ice your feet, particularly immediately after running
- Rest if it becomes too painful to run
- High-arched runners should wear a shoe with soft cushioning in the midsole and ample cushioning in the forefoot

BLISTERS

Blisters are caused by friction when something, usually your shoe, rubs against your skin. The first layer of skin is rubbed so raw that it begins to die and your body causes fluid to build up beneath to protect the tender skin below.

Symptoms

- Rubbing creates an area of irritated skin
- Fluid builds up beneath
- Area becomes sore and expands
- Eventually becomes too painful to run on

Causes

- Improperly fitting shoes
- Socks that create friction

Treatment & Solutions

- Properly fitting shoes
- First-aid treatments such as bandages, tape and Vaseline
- Better-fitting or more cushioned socks, or a second pair
- Rub "Glide" or another blister-preventing lubricant on your feet. These are products made specifically to prevent socks and shoes from rubbing against skin. They are available in running shoe stores and some pharmacies
- Toe socks have a compartment for each toe and provide cushioning
- Silicone toe caps, also available at running shoe stores, fit on your toes and prevent friction
- Many people use duct tape, the incredibly popular tough, gray adhesive stuff that is a fix for every situation known to humankind, to effectively treat blisters (my problem with duct tape is that it isn't porous and therefore it doesn't breathe)

Socks and perspiration can also create problems. The best type of sock is a technical running sock that wicks moisture away from your feet. Cotton socks that retain moisture will result in friction that quickly leads to blistering. Socks that bunch or wear through quickly are blisters waiting to happen.

When blisters are filled with fluid that is not escaping on its own and there is pressure to the touch, you should open them and allow them to drain.

You can cover small blisters with adhesive bandages such as moleskin, but for larger or more serious blisters use Spenco blister patches. This type of bandage was developed during the Vietnam War era to treat burns. It helps keep the area cool and hydrated, and it reduces friction. Some Spenco patches have an adhesive surface that can be applied directly to the skin; with others you'll need to use a porous athletic tape. You should keep a supply of blister remedies in your first-aid kit.

HOW TO TREAT A BLISTER

- *Clean the affected area with hydrogen peroxide*
- *Use a sterile needle*
- *Puncture the blister from the side and allow to drain*
- *If the area looks red and angry, as if infection is setting in, apply an antibiotic ointment*
- *Keep the area clean and apply a bandage*

◆ ◆ ◆

BACK PROBLEMS

Perhaps it's because fitness is simply a good way to keep your back in shape, or maybe it's because runners are better at maintaining an ideal weight and therefore put less strain on their backs—I'm not sure what the reason is—but I see fewer back problems among runners than any other segment of the population I have worked with.

Still, runners are hardly immune from back problems and when they occur they usually bring all workouts to a swift and sometimes prolonged halt.

THINNING OF DISCS

When the discs in our vertebrae become thin it places the bones in close proximity to one another, resulting in pain and restricted movement.

Symptoms

- Lower back pain
- Limited range of motion

Causes

- Natural aging process
- Congenital
- Weak core muscles

Treatment & Solutions

- Chiropractic manipulation
- Stretching back and hamstrings
- Strengthening core and back muscles

SHORT-LEG SYNDROME

Many runners have one leg that is a few millimeters shorter than the other, and this usually won't cause problems. But when the discrepancy amounts to nine millimeters, which is approximately one-third of an inch, over time problems will occur.

Symptoms

- Lower back pain
- Sensation of one foot (heel) striking the ground harder
- Hip or buttock pain

Causes

- Congenital

Treatment & Solutions

- Stretching regimen that emphasizes one side
- Heel lift added to shoe after exact discrepancy is determined
- Chiropractic manipulation
- Exercises to strengthen core and gluteal muscles
- Run with short leg on high side of the road

THINNING OF DISCS

When the discs in our vertebrae become thin it places the bones in close proximity to one another, resulting in pain and restricted movement. The natural aging process is one cause of thinning discs but if it happens gradually and there isn't a sudden change in your running routine, the chances are good your body will adapt and tolerate it.

Birth defects are another cause of back problems. As much as 5% of the population have bones that are not perfectly formed. Again, most won't find it prevents them from running.

The key to longevity for a runner with imperfect discs is a stride that is smooth, not too jarring, and relatively effortless. (*See ChiRunning on page 99.*)

A final cause of disc trouble and lower back pain is tight hamstrings. Tightness in these major muscles in the back of your thighs limits range of motion in the stride and increases pounding.

Whether it's for the health of your knees, Achilles, plantar fascia or your back, a great rule of thumb for runners who work at desks is to get up and stretch every hour. A simple forward bend, to the point where you can feel the stretch begin to burn the backs of your thighs, is a great way to keep your hamstrings from becoming too tight.

SHORT-LEG SYNDROME

A common problem among runners that causes back problems is when one leg is shorter than the other. Many runners have one leg that is a few millimeters shorter than the other, and this usually won't cause problems. But when the discrepancy amounts to nine millimeters, which is approximately one-third of an inch, over time problems will occur.

Some runners with Short-Leg Syndrome say they feel a slight imbalance when they run. Some can see an imbalance when they look at pictures of themselves. Look at a finish line picture of yourself after a long, hard race when fatigue has set in and your form is most likely to have broken down. You may notice several imbalances.

Some runners feel one heel impacting the ground harder than the other, and they can see greater heel wear in one shoe over the other. Some try to correct the problem by running with their short leg toward the middle of the road, which is usually higher, but since it's much safer to run facing traffic, this only works when the right leg is shorter.

The only way to be certain if one leg is shorter and by how much, is to be carefully measured in your health professional's office. If the discrepancy is more than nine millimeters you may benefit from having a lift put in one shoe. Be wary though because a heel lift can lead to a host of serious problems. Hip pain, pain in the side of the knee or back pain can all result from using a heel lift, so you should be evaluated by a health care professional before you begin using one.

*I've given myself
a thousand reasons to
keep running, but it
always comes back to...
self-satisfaction and
a sense of achievement.*

STEVE PREFONTAINE

CHAPTER 4

Safety for Runners

SOMEWHERE IN THE GREAT BEYOND, runners glide along on clouds deliriously unperturbed. But here on planet Earth every car, truck, bus, intersection, driveway, skateboard, bike, pothole, heat wave, cold snap, bumble-bee, yapping terrier and low-hanging branch represents a benign and perhaps beautiful part of our running landscape that can potentially turn troublesome. Running is supposed to be a safe and peaceful sport and most of the time it is. We don't fall down as often as skiers or collide with our fellow competitors like soccer, football or basketball players. But we do find ourselves playing in some less than ideal places, such as in traffic. There is something contradictory in going out on the road to get away from it all. But our safety is mostly in our own hands. We can avoid most of the potential calamities we face by staying alert. Here's what we need to be careful about.

SENSORY PERCEPTION: DON'T GET TRAPPED IN YOUR HEAD

Running is the ultimate in defensive driving. There's no such thing as a fender bender in running. The outcome of an auto vs. pedestrian get-together is entirely predictable.

Since awareness is our best and usually only defense, anything that compromises it is suspect. Take a hard look at habits that lessen your ability to stay awake and avoid trouble. Everything hinges on this question: Are you able to see, hear, smell, taste, touch or otherwise intuit trouble in time to avoid it?

RUNNER'S HIGH

It seems crazy, but at wine tastings people spit out delicious and expensive wine. They do it because they want to stay in control. They want to be able to taste the next wine, or the next seven wines, and they want to be able to drive home.

Like wine, running makes us high. It's a high that doesn't involve ingesting anything, but it's a real high nevertheless, an altered state of consciousness. We all know about endorphins, the hormones in our brains that are released during times of great stress or exertion, including exercise. Endorphins block pain and elevate our sense of pleasure and well-being. "Endorphin" means, "the morphine within." Without endorphins, we'd all be joggers with a one-mile tether.

We like our runner's high. But we have to find the balance that lets us enjoy the release of endorphins without surrendering all our sensory perceptions and our good sense to the experience.

RUN WITH A BUDDY

Running with a partner is a good way to stay grounded. Having someone with you keeps you from floating away.

ESTABLISH CHECK-IN POINTS

Create check-in points on your regular routes as reminders to stay focused. For instance, the mailbox at Union Street is a reminder to be careful at the next intersection. The blue garage under the willow tree reminds me to get up on the sidewalk at the upcoming blind curve.

DON'T TEMPT FATE

Stop at yellow lights even if you think you can dash across in time. Run in place, or run laterally a block and cross at a street where you've got the green light and the "walk" sign. Don't run between parked cars and moving traffic even if you're sure there's plenty of room.

We all need to remember when we are experiencing a runner's high we are more likely to take chances. Endorphins give us the judgment of teenagers; we believe we can do anything and we think we're immortal. What's worse, while we are feeling this way we're not aware of it. We think we're completely normal. To keep ourselves in check, it's smart to be scrupulous about obeying traffic laws.

PLAN YOUR RUN AND RUN YOUR PLAN

If you take your sore plantar fascia out for a 4-miler and two miles into it you feel like you could "run forever," before you veer off onto your 8-mile course, engage your skepticism. Are you fully healed? Have you trained back up to 8-mile territory? Or is that your runner's high talking?

THE HEADPHONE PHENOMENON

I believe that someone who takes up running and runs while listening to her iPod, if she sticks with the sport will eventually find her place in it and the ear buds will fall away. To the novice—and we have all heard them say this—"running is boring." So it may seem. My sense is that a very high percentage of new runners joining the Pasadena Pacers have mp3 players when they come to their first workout. The vast majority will leave them home when they show up for their second or third workout. They soon discover that the road, the rhythms of their own bodies, the music inside their heads and, of course, being with their fellow runners, are all more interesting than the most carefully selected playlist.

The runners who seem most dependent on their iPods are newer runners who quickly become long distance runners and, for whatever reason, find themselves doing long workouts on their own. These are the runners who I feel are at the greatest risk for misadventures.

The danger of headphones is that it robs us of our sense of hearing. If you can't hear a car horn, a revving engine, a barking dog, the shout of a bicyclist or the call of someone passing by, you aren't safe.

Our sense of hearing is too important to sacrifice, regardless of how pleasant it is to listen to music while we run. Experienced runners need to listen to the rhythm of their foot falls and breathing to develop a sense of their pace.

◆ ◆ ◆

TRAFFIC

The first rule of running in traffic is: **don't**. Running trails and other areas, whether designated for recreational use or not, where vehicular traffic is limited or light, are better choices.

Even the guy driving the car with the *share the road* bumper sticker is capable of a mistake some time. Fender benders are as common as spilled milk at daycare, but there is no such thing as a fender bender when there's nothing but running shorts between you and the bumper of a Ford.

GOOD PRACTICES FOR RUNNING IN TRAFFIC

- Run on the left side of the road facing the traffic. If a car is coming at you, you'll have more reaction time if you can see it.
- Running on the left side of the road will also enable you to see oncoming cyclists. Make eye contact with cyclists so they know you see them and aren't going to move into their path. Cyclists are moving too quickly to stop or veer out of your way if you suddenly change course. Even though we're not going that fast, relatively speaking, when we're running in popular spots we do need to pass other runners, and walkers too. A runner darting to the left to pass another runner leaves a cyclist with only bad choices: veer left and risk falling down or being hit by a car coming from behind; or ride into the runner, a collision that is always seen as the cyclist's fault even though it often isn't.
- When running with a partner, only run side by side when there is plenty of room. Never run more than two abreast. When you do run side by side, make sure one runner tucks in behind the other whenever a car approaches.
- Dress to be seen. Wear bright clothing during the day and white and/or reflective clothing at dawn, dusk or night.
- Don't try to beat yellow lights.
- Yield to drivers at intersections where they are making turns.
- Have an escape plan. Make sure you can jump up onto a curb if a car or truck is suddenly coming at you.
- Do not expect a driver to change his direction or path for you.

RUNNING AROUND CURVES AND OVER HILLS

The thing that upsets drivers most about runners is when we surprise them. It gives them an unpleasant jolt of adrenaline similar to when you see police lights flashing in your rear-view mirror. Sometimes they are so startled they feel like they could lose control of their cars. It's an unpleasant and potentially dangerous situation for us both.

Coming around a blind curve or over a hill are two places where it's easy to inadvertently surprise drivers. The important thing is to stay far to the side of the road.

Drivers tend to hug the turn to avoid drifting into the middle of the road. Your place of safety is off the road, even if it means jumping the curb or plunging into some bushes. But if you stray too far into the road and the oncoming car is hugging the turn, you'll have to cross the entire width of the car to get to safety.

That's the situation you want to avoid.

If there is room when you are rounding a blind curve or going over a hill, get completely off the road before you encounter an oncoming car. By listening closely, you might also be able to tell when something is coming your way.

Obviously, curves and hills are two areas where it makes an important difference if you know your route beforehand.

RUNNERS SHOULD BE GOOD NEIGHBORS

When I'm driving and I come upon runners going four abreast chatting away in their private reverie and taking up half the road, I slow to a crawl. I wait until I've got a full clear block in front of me and then I pull far to one side and roll slowly by. I look and wave and the chances are good I know them. It's a small, happy event in my day.

But most motorists are not the founders of running clubs. They are people in a hurry. They probably live on or near the streets we are running through and they think of those streets as their home. They think of us as visitors at best, and nuisances or interlopers at worst. From their point of view, we should be someplace else, on a trail or in a gym or on a treadmill.

At civic meetings you are sure to hear complaints about runners who, to the mind of the aggrieved motorists, were irresponsible, unaware or just plain dopey. Most of these stories include near-misses in which the drivers, invariably non-runners and usually non-athletes, almost hit a runner. Ironically, their ire isn't born of simple impatience, rather, a concern for us.

In any case, except on race day when we've rented it, the road doesn't belong to us and we should act accordingly.

◆ ◆ ◆

CHOOSING A SAFE RUNNING ROUTE

When you get on a plane and go somewhere exciting to run a half marathon, you are the visiting team. The course is unfamiliar, the weather is different and you won't be able to eat your customary pre-race meal.

But training in your neighborhood, you're the home team and you ought to set things up just the way you want them. That means choosing training routes that are varied enough to be interesting, relatively easy on your body, close to home so they're convenient, and they should be safe.

Keep the time of day you'll be running in mind. Parks, neighborhoods and

A Special Note About Cyclists

Cyclists and runners are cousins. When I say, "cyclists," I mean the people with brightly colored jerseys riding thin-tired racing bikes that cost thousands of dollars, for the purpose of getting a serious workout and the enjoyment of their sport. Many of these folks are former runners who because of leg issues simply needed to find a different sport. Others are triathletes who log serious time in running shoes on top of their bike workouts.

If you've ever been on a racing bike on roads with cars, trucks, dogs, runners and baby carriages, you know it's a frightening proposition. We runners are plodding along, most of us, at 5 to 7 mph, with our feet barely leaving the ground. Cyclists are going 15 to 20 mph or faster (they'll go 30 to 40 mph down hills), on machines that, without the balancing skills of their riders, will fall over in one second. Oftentimes they ride elbow to elbow in a group and if one of them goes down they might as well throw a party in the emergency room because that's where several of them are headed.

The margin for error when riding a racing bike is very small. So when you hear a cyclist call out a loud and possibly rude-sounding warning as he or she speeds toward you from behind, know that these are the concerns running through his mind.

The best practice when riding in an area populated by cyclists is to stay to the side and let them have the lane between the far edge of the road and the middle, where the vehicular traffic is. Run single file, don't make sudden left-right movements and make sure you can hear (no earphones) and are listening for them zipping up from behind.

even some streets change their character according to the time of day. For instance, a street that runs past a school might be completely free of traffic at 7 a.m. but jammed with buses and minivans at 3:15 in the afternoon. A park full of nannies and toddlers at 10 a.m. might feel dark and frightening after dark.

RECREATIONAL AREAS

Look first for a recreational area with a path or trail specifically designated for runners. This is where you'll most likely find a place that is:

- Free from vehicular traffic
- Has a smooth path with a soft surface
- Adequate lighting
- Water
- Other runners and/or people exercising

RESIDENTIAL NEIGHBORHOODS

A second choice is residential neighborhoods. Look for ones that border on recreational sites such as major parks, golf courses or high school athletic fields. Seek out these attributes:

- Wide streets (you should be able to pass a parked car without running in the direct path of an oncoming vehicle)
- A low speed limit (speed bumps also help)
- Light traffic
- Adequate lighting
- Smooth pavement that isn't filled with cracks and potholes

RESEARCH & RESOURCES

- Drive your route before you run it. See firsthand how well lit it is, how much traffic it has and what it feels like at different times of day. You can also measure it and note mile markers.
- Websites like usatf.org/routes (the USA Track & Field site), mapmyrun. com and runtheplanet.com have databases of routes mapped by other runners. The sites include mile markers, comments from the runners who posted them and other information like where you can find water and public rest rooms along the way. The USATF site has more than 300,000 such postings, so it's likely you can find routes in your neighborhood, or you can create your own. The sites have mapping programs enabling you to draw your own routes. They will automatically insert your mile markers for you.

WEATHER

One of the great things about running is it keeps us in contact with the natural world. Dr. George Sheehan, the cardiologist, philosopher, writer (*Running and Being*, 1978) and patron saint of running, often quoted Emerson as saying, in order to be a good human being, "first, be a good animal." A willingness to brave the elements, we spoiled Californians need to be reminded, is part of that.

It's also important to push the envelope of reason once in a while. As you know, I believe in running at least once a year in the rain (*see pages 74-75*), and also—at least here in California—on the coldest day of the year, which might mean temperatures in the high 30s. No big deal for a Minnesotan.

That said, taking on extreme weather with raw determination but without precautions isn't the answer.

RUNNING IN THE COLD

During a long, cold winter run, limit the distance you will travel from home or other places you know you can retreat to if you get in trouble. You can do this by running shorter loops—for instance, instead of running a 6-mile loop, run a 2-mile loop and go around three times. Finally, consider carrying a cell phone. The following preperation steps and cold weather gear will help you be ready for sub-freezing temperatures and/or wind chill factors.

- Know the conditions you'll be running in. Don't assume conditions won't change during your run. Will the sun set? Is there a chance the wind will pick up?
- Include the wind chill in the temperature you are dressing for.
- Some 30% to 40% of your body's heat loss can escape through your hands and feet, so definitely wear a hat and gloves. Don't wait for bitter cold to start wearing them. Elite marathoners wear hats and gloves when temperatures are in the 50s, and sometimes 60s.
- Keep your hands warm and dry with two layers. The first layer should be a wicking material that keeps the perspiration away from your skin. The outer layer should also shed moisture while keeping warmth inside, and it should screen out the wind.
- Your hat should cover your ears as well as the entire surface of your head.
- Wear three layers on your upper body: the first should be a high-tech fabric that wicks away moisture. The second should be a material that keeps warm air close to your body but doesn't trap or hold on to moisture. The outside layer should screen the wind and keep snow from melting and penetrating to your inside layers.

- Running pants should keep snow off your legs and hold in warmth. In extreme cold you may need a second layer of a fabric such as silk or Capilene® that wicks moisture while retaining body heat.
- Don't wear cotton. It soaks up moisture and holds it like a cold sponge.
- Use petroleum jelly and/or a lip balm such as ChapStick to insulate your lips, nose and the tips of your ears from the wind.

RISKS OF RUNNING IN THE COLD

There are two dangers to running in cold weather: *frostbite* and *hypothermia*.

Frostbite

Frostbite is the freezing of skin and possibly the underlying tissue. Hands, feet, nose and ears are the main areas of concern because they are the parts of the body furthest from the heart and have the weakest circulation. Prevent frostbite by wearing layers. The outer layer should be of a material that screens out wind.

Monitor these areas on a long, cold run. If your extremities feel a little numb at first but they warm up as your core heats up, you're fine. But if the numbness and a slight burning sensation give way to no feeling and no pain, this could be frostbite taking hold. Other signs of frostbite are hard, cold, pale patches that will eventually swell and redden.

If you think you are suffering frostbite on a run:
- Stop running and get to a warm place out of the wind.
- Warm your affected areas by wrapping them in extra clothing. While still in the cold, put your hands in your armpits.
- Don't rub a frostbitten area. Rubbing can damage frozen skin.
- Warm up as soon as possible. The determining factor in the amount of damage done by frostbite is not how cold a part of your body becomes, but how long it remains frozen.
- Warm your core with a hot, non-caffeinated, non-alcoholic drink.
- If numbness persists, seek emergency care.

Hypothermia

Hypothermia is when your body is losing heat faster than it can produce it, and your body temperature falls below 95° F (normal is 98.6° F).

On a long run on a bitter cold day it's conceivable you could run out of your depth and find yourself weakened a long way from home or safety. Remember, your body is working harder than normal when you are out in bitter cold. It takes energy to keep your temperature elevated dozens of degrees higher than

Why We Run in the Rain (and Other Bad Weather)

For nearly 15 years, the Pasadena Pacers have run every Saturday morning at 7 a.m., without missing a single Saturday. Since we live in California, we do not have to contend with blizzards, bitter cold, tornadoes or hurricanes. But we have run when wildfires were burning nearby, when mudslides were threatening to fall upon us, when it was much colder than we would have liked (in the 30s) and most definitely we have run in the rain.

When training for races, it's important to be a little unreasonable because during the race, your reasonableness will definitely be questioned. If it rains, if it's brutally hot, if you encounter more hills than you planned on, or if you just don't feel right, you will come up against the temptation to quit. What then? When your training includes periods of being unreasonable, instances of challenging and overcoming that reasonable voice inside that whispers, "This isn't really necessary," you'll be prepared and you'll persevere.

Here is something I wrote to the Pacers in response to a question from a newcomer on whether or not we run in the rain. It's become our manifesto on running in bad weather:

> *We are the Pacers and we always run, rain or shine.*
> *There are two days of the year when we always run: on the coldest day and on the rainiest day. This is based on the*

principle that in order to be extraordinary, one should never be reasonable. Going into agreement with mediocrity allows you to sleep in on Saturday, take a day off when you are feeling uninspired and stay indoors when it rains.

No measure of greatness was ever achieved by being reasonable. Be audacious, get unreasonable and live outrageously because that's who we are—by God, we are the Pacers!

Bold words are wonderful, but does the strategy work? Yes, it does. The inaugural Pasadena Marathon was run in February of 2009, largely in a driving rain. Two dozen Pacers started and finished that race. And the L.A. Marathon of 2011 was run in a rainstorm that dumped five inches of precipitation on some sections of southern California as the race was run. All 60 Pacers who started that race finished, each one a champion.

Yes, we are the Pacers and we run in the rain!

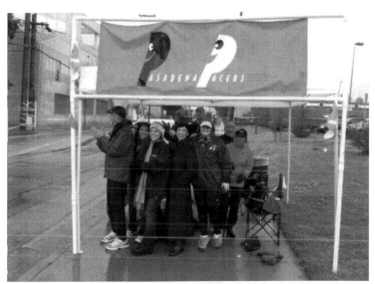

FOUNDER STEVE AND FELLOW PACERS SUPPORT PARTICIPANTS OF THE RAINY, WET 2011 LOS ANGELES MARATHON. PHOTO ROBIN SMITH

the surrounding air. Meanwhile, you're still expending the energy necessary to cover the miles. Footing in winter weather is typically more difficult, adding another stressor to your system and there may also be wind to contend with.

The longer you are exposed to extreme cold, the more likely you are to develop hypothermia. On a ten-degree day with sub-zero wind chill, one runner dashing through a four-mile run in under 30 minutes might fare well, whereas the runner pacing 11-minute miles is out in the cold 50% longer and therefore faces greater risk.

Symptoms of hypothermia include shivering, impaired speech, confusion and poor decision-making.

RUNNING IN THE HEAT

A wise, old runner who preferred running in the cold to running in the heat, said, "You can always put more clothes on, but there comes a point where you can't take any more off."

HYPERTHERMIA AND HEAT STROKE

Hyperthermia is when body temperature rises too high because the body is absorbing more heat than it can dissipate. Hyperthermia can lead to heat stroke, where the body temperature rises, potentially to 104 degrees or higher. A person experiencing heat stroke may stop sweating and become confused or even unconscious. The skin becomes red, hot and dry.

Heat stroke is a medical emergency. Heat stroke victims should be taken to an emergency room or urgent care center so they can receive intravenous fluids and be cooled via a medical process. In the meantime, victims should rest in the coolest place available. Apply ice packs or cool water to the groin, underarms and neck.

HYDRATION

The human body is composed of about 70% water so we run on fluid. Not having enough water—and that is the greatest challenge associated with running in hot weather—will clearly affect performance. You won't be able to run as long or as fast and your chances of injury and/or illness skyrocket.

Besides fatigue, dehydration will also lead to muscle cramping including, potentially, the severe type of cramps that can take weeks to fully release and meanwhile make running impossible. There is nothing worse than waiting all winter for better running weather only to have a calf muscle or hamstring seize up on the first hot day of summer.

Back in the dark ages, before about 1980, most athletic coaches limited water intake during workouts because of the misguided fear that fluid sloshing in stomachs would lead to nausea. What actually happened was that athletes became dehydrated and suffered heat stroke. Indeed, a number of high school kids training in brutal late-summer heat became seriously ill and a few even died.

Today we have the science of "hydration," which means maintaining a balanced amount of fluid in our systems—neither too much, nor too little. How much fluid you should drink, and what kind, depends on the heat, humidity, duration of your run, how hard you are working and your individual body chemistry.

The rule of thumb is, drink 16 ounces for every pound you lose during your workout. Another general yardstick says the average runner should drink six to eight ounces every 20 minutes during a workout on a hot day.

This is all well and good, but you should go beyond these generalities and learn your body's particular needs. To start, weigh yourself naked before and after a series of workouts. What you are looking for is approximately how much weight you will lose during a given workout, depending on the temperature, duration and other variables. If you lose two pounds during your run, you know 32 ounces was the appropriate amount you should have consumed while you were on the course. Take that information into account on subsequent workouts.

Once you get the calibrations figured out, your goal is to drink enough during your run so that regardless of the heat, the duration and the intensity, you don't lose more than 1% of your body weight.

It is possible to drink too much, particularly if you are drinking only water. Water can dilute the electrolytes in your system and cause problems, sometimes severe, if the levels of certain minerals fall too low. And yes, the old-fashioned concerns about a belly full of water causing stomach problems are valid. It is better to take frequent sips than to hold off and guzzle.

It's also important to show up for a workout or a race properly hydrated, rather than waiting until you are out on the course to start drinking. A good guideline for knowing you are staying properly hydrated throughout the week, is when you urinate several times a day and the color of your urine is like straw or pale lemonade.

BRINGING WATER WITH YOU

During a properly organized race, drinking three to four ounces every mile or so will be simple since volunteers will hand you cups on the course. But during workouts, especially those lasting more than 30 minutes, you need to carry your own fluids.

Lightweight belts with Velcro closures and carrying slots for two to four plastic bottles, capable of holding up to 16 ounces each, are now readily available. Definitely get one and use it. The benefits of being properly hydrated far outweigh the temporary inconvenience of becoming accustomed to wearing a belt. (Most belts also contain a handy pocket for keys, money, identification, a cell phone, blister first-aid, etc., thus solving several problems at once.) If you need more fluids, you can try a wearable hydration pack, or bladder, capable of holding up to 100 ounces. You wear these bladder systems like a backpack and drink the fluids through a hose that reaches over your shoulder.

RUNNING IN POLLUTED AIR

On Sunday, November 16, 2008, the organizers of the inaugural Pasadena Marathon postponed the race because several wildfires in the outlying parts of Los Angeles County had filled the air with ash and smoke. Everyone was cautioned not to exert themselves and people with breathing problems were told to stay indoors. Breathing as deeply as we do when running was obviously unsafe.

Many runners were upset at the decision and at first glance, that's understandable. Some 8,000 runners had registered, paid and trained for the race. Many had traveled great distances and now they were in Pasadena ready to run. Hundreds of us had worked for years to persuade local officials and business people to back the race. A lot of money had been raised. Despite high hopes, no one had any idea if another date could be found when the inaugural race could go off. There was a lot of pressure to run.

But in the end, there was no other decision. No matter where you went in town, it smelled like you were standing right next to the grill at a very large barbecue. Light flakes of ash the size of small grains of rice, dirty white in color, were falling from the sky. We woke up on marathon morning to find our cars covered with ash like a light dusting of snow.

Wildfire smoke is a rare and extreme condition that affects a minority of runners. What we should all be cautious about is everyday pollutants caused by industries and traffic, especially in urban areas. Athletes take in an estimated 10 to 20 times as much air as sedentary people and we breathe that air more deeply into our lungs. We know that particles of pollutants, many of them too small to see without an electron microscope, lodge deep in our lungs where it's beyond our physiological ability to cleanse them. What are affected are our alveoli, the tiny, grape-like clusters of blood vessels deep within our lungs that can become damaged when particles are trapped there. It's not just lung damage that is at stake. Recent treadmill studies with runners breathing piped-in polluted air showed impairment of blood vessels, including the kinds of constriction that can damage the heart.

The three pollutants we are most concerned about are ozone (O_3) which forms when sunlight reacts with tailpipe emissions and is therefore a bigger problem in Phoenix than London; sulfur dioxide (SO_2), which comes out of industrial smokestacks; and carbon monoxide (CO), the most common urban pollutant, which is created by burning fossil fuels. Carbon monoxide actually attaches to hemoglobin, the protein in red blood cells that carries oxygen around the body, and that can have a brutal effect on your blood's ability to deliver oxygen to muscles.

The quality of city air changes according to the time of day, the degree of industrial activity, traffic level, proximity to high traffic areas and the temperature. Summer heat makes everything worse. Inversions that trap polluted air over a city are especially bad for runners. It's a rule of thumb that when you can see the air (or smell it) it's probably too dirty to run in.

Unfortunately, we don't have a handy measurement we can point to and advise, "Above this threshhold, you have to come inside on the treadmill." Even the day the inaugural Pasadena Marathon was canceled, there were no widely circulated parameters officials were able to point to as justification for their decision.

The Environmental Protection Agency (EPA) produces a daily report using an "air quality index" *(see it at airnow.gov)* that runs from 0 to 500 with anything over 100 designated as unhealthy for some people. The criteria used for arriving at the scores is complicated, to say the least, and while it is widely distributed, it hasn't yet been broadly adopted as the comprehensible standard, probably because so few people base their behavior on what it says. But you can go to the site, plug in your zip code and get a reading that's of some general use. Local agencies might provide more detailed information depending on where you live.

The inaugural Pasadena Marathon was rescheduled and run on March 22, 2009. It was a great race, much of it in the rain.

GOOD PRACTICES FOR AIR QUALITY AND RUNNING

- Find a local source you can use to check the air quality in your neighborhood and consult it regularly.
- Pay particular attention to air quality if you live in or near a major urban area; also if you live near a place with heavy traffic, such as a highway or an airport.
- Scrutinize the air more closely on very hot days.
- Do your best to create an indoor alternative where you can run on bad air days.
- Run inside or take the day off if you can see, smell or taste the pollution in the air.

CRIME AND OTHER DANGERS

One of the first books ever written about running, years before the first boom, was *On the Run from Dogs and People* by Hal Higdon. The title itself is a reminder that many of us, at one time or another, have had to flee some danger while out on a run.

MUGGERS

Among the Pasadena Pacers whose running histories I'm familiar with, I can quickly count hundreds of years of running experience without anyone having been accosted on the road. I've always wondered about the mind of a mugger who would attack someone who was not carrying a purse or a briefcase and apparently doesn't even have any pockets. Mugger's logic aside, runners are attacked from time to time. Sexual assaults of women are a particular concern. It's up to each of us to minimize the dangers to ourselves and our fellow runners, and here's how:

- Choose running routes that are well lit and populated. Stay away from secluded areas. This can be challenging since many of us have solitary natures and enjoy getting away. I get it. No one wants to run at the mall a week before Christmas. But please put your safety first. If you run in the park early Saturday morning, you can enjoy solitude and safety at the same time; running in a secluded place on Thursday night at 10 p.m. is a different matter.
- Run with a buddy or a group.
- Carry a whistle and be prepared to use it.
- Carry a cell phone.
- If you have safety concerns about a particular route, even mild ones, but you're not willing to abandon the route, run through the sketchy sections of the route first when you are fresh. Don't save the questionable section for last when you may or may not have a kick left.
- Think through every route and know which way you would run at any given point if you were approached. In the unlikely event you someday find yourself being chased, which way you run in those first moments will make a big difference. Be aware of which is the shortest distance to safety. Run toward the busy street, not the river.

DOGS

If you run long enough, often enough and in enough different places, sooner or later it will happen. You will be chased by a dog.

Let's all agree that the vast majority of dog owners are responsible citizens who keep their dogs on leashes or safely in their yards behind secure fences. I mean no offense to dogs or their owners (I have three of my own) but there is a significant minority of folks who are sometimes lax in the care of their animals. Sometimes those animals go unattended and are free to come after runners.

Some people ask, "So what?" Dogs are territorial, barking and chasing is what they naturally do, they are not running through our neighborhoods, rather, it is we who are infringing on their turf. All well and good, except most of us don't want to be bitten.

According to the Centers for Disease Control and Prevention, dogs bite more than 4 million people per year, nearly a million of them require medical attention and 31,000 need reconstructive surgery. Let's not be among them.

- If there is an aggressive dog on any of your regular routes, change the route. Simply run down a different street. Even if your barker is inside a fence that is always secure, why run the risk that on the 99th time you run past, he's able to get out?
- If you are chased, stop running. Instinctively, dogs chase things that run.
- Face the dog so it doesn't appear you are fleeing, but don't assume a threatening pose. Most dog experts suggest you not make eye contact.
- From the dog's point of view, you are invading his turf. To remedy the situation, walk away in the opposite direction. Typically, when a dog barks and chases us he is inside a fence. While it's annoying, it's not sufficient reason to break off course, and we continue running the length of the yard. But if the dog gets loose, change course immediately. If it means crossing the street, by all means be careful, but know that the dog is less likely to follow you that way than if you continue laterally across or past his turf.
- If you lose the race and the dog is close enough to bite you, stop and stand still. In a calm but firm voice, tell the dog, "No."

◆ ◆ ◆

IDENTIFICATION

An accident that would render you unable to speak while you are out on the roads is unlikely, but it could happen. One estimate is that 500,00 people per year in the U.S. are taken to emergency rooms unconscious. Car accidents, violent attacks, heart attack, heat stroke and sudden, unexplained medical incidents

Why It's Smart to Run with a Partner or Group

- Keep one another alert to traffic and other potential hazards.

- Reduces the likelihood of being approached or harassed by potential troublemakers, be they two-legged or four-legged.

- Someone can provide assistance in the event of injury—four miles home through the snow with a twisted ankle is no fun.

- Motivation. You are more likely to show up and stay with it if someone else is involved.

- Conversation keeps us all going.

- Pacesetting. Running with someone at or just a little bit ahead of your accustomed pace is a great way to improve your training.

- Running with partners forces you to vary your routes.

- Running dissolves the social barriers we unwittingly build around ourselves. When we break down these barriers it's much easier to bond and create friendships. One lesson that's been learned and enjoyed thousands of times among our running group, the Pasadena Pacers, is that every person is interesting once you get to know them. We each have a terrific story. Despite our social defenses, we all want to discover the person running next to us, and be discovered too.

are the main culprits.

Without dwelling on the likelihood of any of these or other unpredictable calamities happening, it's simply a good idea to carry identification when out on the roads. Shoe pockets and identification bands that strap around your wrist or ankle, both with your information printed on them, are readily available and affordable (under $20). Cheaper still, print your information on a card, laminate it and carry it in your pocket.

If you carry a cell phone, make sure you have an ICE number (In Case of Emergency) in your directory. Your runner's ID should include:

- Your name
- Emergency contact names and phone numbers
- Special medical information such as allergies, conditions or special needs
- Blood type
- Primary care physician's name and number

*Play not only keeps us
young but also maintains
our perspective about the
relative seriousness of things.
Running is play, for even if
we try hard to do well at it,
it is a relief from everyday cares.*

JIM FIXX

CHAPTER 5

A Matter of Heart

RUNNING IS GOOD FOR YOU. Never doubt it. But there is something that causes people to question the safety and wisdom of running, and that is when they see or hear about someone collapsing during or after a race and dying. It shocks us all. As many writers have pointed out, the first paragraph of the news coverage inevitably includes the word, "ironic." It doesn't make sense. If running is so good for us, how can it kill someone?

The answer, of course, is that running doesn't kill people. Marathon and half-marathoners who have heart attacks are almost always people who have brought their medical problems to the race with them. Yes, strenuous exercise—any kind of exercise—can trigger a heart attack, but not in healthy people. A fascinating study showed heart attack deaths spiking after a heavy snowfall because a preponderance of people who had heart disease, but didn't know it, put themselves through heavy workouts shoveling snow. Afterward, however, heart attack deaths fell sharply for a period of time because there were relatively few people left who were unknowingly sick and on the verge of having a heart attack. The next snowfall and spate of shoveling didn't claim nearly as many lives.

One of the dangers of heart disease is that it's insidious: you can have heart problems without knowing it. Too often, the first symptom of heart disease is a heart attack.

WHY RUNNERS HAVE HEART ATTACKS

When a runner collapses during or soon after a race it is usually for one of two reasons. Younger runners, 30 to 35 or younger, who suffer heart attacks almost always have a condition called hypertrophic cardiomyopathy. This is a thickening in the wall of the heart muscle that leads to an enlarged heart. An enlarged heart is a confusing concept because bigger muscles are usually better muscles, and athletes' muscles, including the heart, usually are bigger and stronger performers. If you've run several marathons your heart is probably significantly larger and more efficient than that of a sedentary person. However, a heart that becomes enlarged not from exercise but from struggling to cope with a congenital abnormality, such as hypertrophic cardiomyopathy, is actually weaker and more prone to fail. When these hearts fail their ability to maintain a consistent rhythm is often the first function to go, and the distress can escalate so quickly that death quickly follows. When you hear about a 30-year-old runner who had a heart attack at a race, it was likely caused by this or one of several similar, complicated congenital heart diseases.

Runners over 35 who have heart attacks almost always suffered for some time from coronary artery disease, but didn't know it. In a landmark article in *Runners World* (December 2008) by Amby Burfoot on heart attacks and runners, heart specialist Paul Thompson, M.D., one of the world's leading experts on heart disease and exercise, dicussed what happens when a runner has coronary artery disease:

The disease is caused by cholesterol deposits in the arteries that supply the heart with blood. Thompson described these vessels as like a garden hose with a modest flow of water moving through it. When you begin to run, blood flows more rapidly through your arteries and the volume increases. It's like the flow of water through the garden hose increasing dramatically. The hose begins to twist and flail; you've felt this when you've held a garden hose, Thompson said, or seen it when firefighters have to brace themselves to control a high-pressure hose.

If you have a cholesterol deposit in one of your coronary arteries, this flexing and bending of the vessel can crack the deposit open and break it loose. Your blood mixes with the cholesterol to form a clot that blocks the artery and in a few minutes you're in real trouble.

THE DEATH OF JIM FIXX

The original and quintessential runner's heart attack took the life of Jim Fixx, the celebrated author of the bestseller, *The Complete Book of Running*. Fixx was a national figure and the unofficial leader of the first running boom who died while running in Vermont on July 20, 1984, at age 52. An autopsy showed Fixx had significant blockages in all three coronary arteries. In recounting Fixx's final days, his family realized there had been warning signs: Fixx had awakened one night in a cold sweat, barely able to breathe; on a run with his son, he had to stop uncharacteristically after a half mile as he was experiencing breathlessness, which he attributed vaguely to allergies; and he had tightness in his upper arm. But Fixx stoically discounted these symptoms, not to mention his heredity: his father had his first heart attack at 37 and died at 41.

The sight or simply the prospect of a runner collapsing is as sobering as it is sad. There is the automatic urge to tie the two together—"running" and "collapse," as cause and effect. Then there is the ever-present whisper suggesting, "This running is too much effort, it's not worth it. Let's just head for the couch, the clicker and the bag of chips." What better anti-motivation than the prospect of a heart attack?

But of course, none of it is true. Jim Fixx's most remembered statement is probably, "Running may not add years to your life, but it definitely adds life to your years." Today we know running probably does add years to your life, and it probably added several years to Jim Fixx's. When he started running at the age of 36, he was more than 50 pounds overweight and a heavy smoker. His genes, together with that kind of lifestyle, made Fixx a bad bet to outlive his dad. But his family was told by the medical examiner after the autopsy, that strengthening his heart muscle by running, probably extended Jim Fixx's life by eight to ten years.

OVERWHELMING ODDS IN YOUR FAVOR

Several studies of runners dying during or just after marathons have put the odds at somewhere between one in 100,000 and one in 200,000. Meanwhile, your chances of dying in a motor-vehicle accident at some point in your life are one in 85. Here are some other approximate odds of dying in a given year based on statistics from the National Safety Council:

Riding in a car	*1 in 6,500*
Accidental fall	*1 in 15,500*
Drowning	*1 in 85,000*
Caught in a fire	*1 in 90,000*
Choking on food	*1 in 325,000*
Hit by lightning	*1 in 6.5 million*

As Dr. Paul Thompson sums it up, "If you want to live a long, vigorous life, you should do an hour of moderate exercise a day. If your only goal is to survive the next hour of your life, you should get into bed—alone."

There is a difference between saying that the chances that someone will die running a marathon are one in, let's say, 150,000, versus saying that your chances of dying in a race are one in 150,000. What the statistics actually mean, are that if 150,000 runners are running a marathon on a particular day, one person will have a fatal heart attack. But since we know that this unlucky imaginary runner probably has a pre-existing heart condition, the question is not, "Will you be the unfortunate runner who is randomly stricken?" Rather, the question is, "Are you the runner walking up to the starting line who has latent, advanced heart disease?"

Heart disease is so tricky that there is the possibility, although very small, that you could have your heart examined, pass the tests with flying colors, and yet develop heart disease soon thereafter. Nevertheless, there are many things we can do to take that unvarnished one in 150,000 risk and make it more like one in a million.

SEVEN WAYS TO MINIMIZE YOUR RISK OF HEART TROUBLE
Genetics
Pay attention to your family history. If you have parents, grandparents, uncles and aunts with heart trouble, or who died from heart attacks, you are more likely to be affected.

Know the Warning Signs
The classic warning signs of heart disease are:
- persistent shortness of breath
- pain and a tight feeling in the chest
- feeling of heart racing
- unusual and persistent fatigue

Get a Stress Test
Tests that create an image of your heart, and others that record your heart's rhythm can tell cardiologists volumes about the health of your heart.

Know and Maintain Your Cholesterol Levels
Cholesterol leads to plaque buildup in your coronary arteries. A simple blood test can tell your cholesterol level and while that won't tell you about potential blockages in your arteries, high cholesterol is the first step in the wrong direction.

Know and Maintain Your Blood Pressure

High blood pressure is a leading contributor to heart disease. Fortunately, it's one of the simplest readings to take, and as a runner you are way ahead in terms of controlling your blood pressure.

Race-day Protocol

Many heart experts recommend following these two tips on race day to reduce your chance of heart trouble.

- Drink less than 200 mg of caffeine. Caffeine can play a factor in disrupting the heart's ability to beat rhythmically. (Starbucks lists its tall size coffee as having 260 mg of caffeine, and a single shot as containing 75 mg.)
- Maintain your speed as you finish your race rather than running all out. Some studies have shown more heart attacks occur in the final mile of the race and some heart doctors suspect that accelerating at the end of a long, grueling and relatively slow race could be the cause (for those with latent heart disease).

When in Doubt, Check It Out

Most heart attack sufferers, upon reflecting, realize there were warning signs they ignored, or noticed but discounted. In the long run, no pun intended, it makes more sense if you have suspicions, to have yourself examined. The good news is that most types of heart disease are treatable, but it's best if they're detected prior to the crisis of a heart attack. So don't ignore the feedback your body gives you. Listen to your body and learn to interpret its signs, and then give your body what it needs.

BE READY TO HELP OTHERS

There is one more important thing you can do to chip away at the risk of death from heart disease—not your death, but the potential deaths of others—and that is to learn CPR (cardiopulmonary resuscitation). Not everyone who has a heart attack dies, in fact, far from it. The most important factor is how long it takes for medical help to arrive. Because medical help is so prevalent along courses, fewer than half the heart attacks suffured during marathons are fatal. One cardiologist quipped that a marathon is a great place to have a heart attack. You can be trained in CPR any number of places in your community. The courses usually take less than a day and are often free. Hospitals, YMCAs and your local health department are three great places to find a course.

The good we do for ourselves as runners far outweighs the risk of harm. In theory, you could be in a car accident, in which it would be better to be thrown from the vehicle than held in place by your seat belt. But we still wear seat belts. So it is with running. Out of some 30 million runners in the United States, a couple hundred could be courting some degree of serious risk. But the rest of us only have to deal with occasional, relatively minor injuries.

When it's pouring
rain and you're bowling
along through the wet,
there's satisfaction in
knowing you're out there
and the others aren't.

PETER SNELL

CHAPTER 6

Cross-Training

A LACK OF CROSS-TRAINING has been the downfall of many a distance runner. There is a lot of truth in the idea that to be a good runner you have to run. The problem is that running does not train every muscle in your body. I wouldn't say that by having running as your only form of exercise you are completely neglecting any part of your body. I don't think running leaves any part of the body as weak as if you were completely sedentary. But the disparity in the degree to which certain muscles are trained can become a problem. Nature may abhor a vacuum, but she's not too kind about imbalance either, and in athletics, any imbalance left alone for too long usually results in a problem.

For instance, running trains the tops and the outside of the quadriceps beautifully, but the inside or medial quadriceps to a much lesser extent. The result can be improper tracking of the knee joint, leading to a variety of knee problems. Consequently, workouts that strengthen the inner thighs are good for runners.

◆ ◆ ◆

TIPS FOR A SUCCESSFUL CROSS-TRAINING REGIMEN

COMBAT BOREDOM

Not every runner is a fanatic and not every fanatical runner is 100% enthused with running all the time. When I treat injured runners, I sometimes wonder if the cause of the injury wasn't simply that the body, or the psyche, simply needed a break. We are human beings, not machines, and our imaginations need stimulation. Just like it's a good idea to go somewhere you've never been before at least once a year, so it's good for athletes to try a new, or at least different form of exercise every so often. Cross training makes dashing through your favorite running route that much sweeter.

DON'T SLACK OFF

"Cross-training" is not Latin for "day off." Many runners fear that they will lose fitness by exchanging a running day for cross-training. That will become a self-fulfilling prophesy when you don't take the workout seriously. Just because you are not running doesn't mean you shouldn't be working hard. You will continue to build fitness during your cross-training workouts by keeping your heart rate at or above 70% of your maximum (calculate your maximum by subtracting your age from 220).

BEWARE OF OVERTRAINING

Runners who commit to cross-training but aren't willing to trade in one of their running workouts face the danger of overtraining. It's interesting to note that if you tried to add another running workout to a full regimen, your body might simply reject it in the form of brutally sore muscles. But if you add a cross-training workout in which you are stressing different muscles, you might be able to get away without any added soreness, only to have your body talk back to you in the form of fatigue. How can you tell? One sign is if you hit a plateau in your running performances. Another is if, instead of waking up sore but rejuvenated the morning after a good workout, you simply feel fatigued. A third sign is an elevated morning heart rate. (Check your morning heart rate periodically so you have a baseline as your running career progresses.)

UPPER-BODY STRENGTH

You don't need to be able to bench press your weight in order to finish a marathon. But having some strength in your upper body helps maintain integrity of running form, especially when fatigue is setting in. Spend a few minutes at the finish line of a marathon or half-marathon some time and you will appreciate the importance of upper-body strength for runners. The most fatigued runners are so slumped over it's hard to believe they are moving forward. The complications it presents for their body mechanics are bad enough, but the worst consequence is how hard it becomes to breathe. In contrast, the runners who are still upright, their chests open, have a much easier time getting air into their lungs.

◆ ◆ ◆

GOOD CROSS-TRAINING OPTIONS FOR RUNNERS

SWIMMING

It doesn't get any more "low-impact" than swimming. You can't beat the weight-lessness of water when you are recovering from an injury. Consequently, the pool is the first stop for runners looking to stay in shape while they heal and before they are ready to get back on the roads. Because it won't put any stress on your legs, is a great aerobic workout and will help tone your upper body, swimming is a great cross-training choice. If you mix in the breaststroke, with its frog-like kick, you'll get a good inner-thigh workout that is great for balancing the strength of your quadriceps and heading off knee trouble.

CYCLING

Like swimming, cycling also provides a great aerobic workout while placing minimal stress on leg muscles, particularly compared with running. You don't get much of an upper-body workout. Cycling works your inner thighs more than running. If you are a runner with no cycling experience taking it up for cross-training purposes, have someone who knows cycling give you an orientation on how, where and when to ride safely. For safety, you can't beat the stationary bike.

ELLIPTICAL TRAINER

This machine can provide a total-body workout, including the upper body, if you use the poles to work your arms. The oval-like rotation your feet make, in the shape of an ellipse, and hence the name, works many of the same muscles you fire when you run. There is very low stress placed on your legs. If you run the machine backward, you can work your gluteal muscles, but there is no way to focus on your inner quads.

ROWING

There aren't many people who have access to some form of open-water rowing, but most gyms offer rowing machines. This is another exercise form that completely avoids pounding your legs. It will give you an excellent cardiovascular workout. It's great for strengthening quads, hips, gluteals and quadriceps. It 's a very good upper body workout.

NORDIC TRACK/CROSS-COUNTRY SKIING

A great workout that combines cardiovascular intensity with upper-body strengthening, and also works many leg muscles that are not highly developed through running. This is a good choice for runners looking to cross-train, but it requires some coordination and it will take you some time to learn proper form.

ROLLERBLADING

Rollerblading exaggerates the running form. It's a great quadriceps and gluteal workout, and it is an aerobic workout too. It's one of the best cross-training choices if you are concerned about ITBS.

*Your goals must come from
your body and from your
present reality, not from other
people's idea of what's cool...
Let your goals be an expression
of who you are, not something
that will impress someone
or earn praise.*

DANNY DREYER

CHAPTER 7

ChiRunning

CHIRUNNING IS A new approach to running developed in the last ten years by Danny Dreyer, an ultra-marathoner and serious, longtime student of T'ai Chi, the Chinese martial art form.

T'ai Chi stresses balance and alignment, and the idea of working in harmony with natural forces to create powerful, fluid movements. Danny believed he could apply these principles to running in a way that would improve biomechanics and help us run with less pounding and less effort. His ambition, and it's a mighty one, is to revolutionize running to the point where it's no longer a sport with a high rate of injuries.

As he puts it, "ChiRunning combines the inner focus and flow of T'ai Chi with the power and energy of running to create a revolutionary running form and philosophy that takes the pounding, pain and potential damage out of the sport...(It) turns running into a safe and effective lifelong program for health, fitness and well-being."

At first glance, I thought Danny's ideas were hooey. We Homo sapiens have been running since the days when if we didn't catch what we were chasing, we starved. It didn't seem likely that someone had "discovered" something new about running.

But then I read his book, *ChiRunning: A Revolutionary Approach to Effortless, Injury-free Running* (Simon & Schuster, 2004), and, more importantly, I met Kathy Greist, one of the first people Danny certified to teach ChiRunning. I didn't seek out Kathy. Rather, she showed up one Saturday morning at a regular Pasadena Pacers workout. She wasn't there to teach or evangelize, just to run with us.

Despite my skepticism, I was curious. Kathy had a beautiful running form that indeed looked, if not effortless, then at least smooth and easy. She explained that ChiRunning is simply "teaching a biomechanically correct running form that is in line with the laws of physics." That grabbed me. I've always been a fan of working with, rather than against, the laws of physics.

We soon asked Kathy to present ChiRunning seminars for the Pacers. Many of our members turned out and reported feeling more comfortable with their strides. I was one of them.

What I like about ChiRunning most of all is that it goes right to the heart of the challenge every runner faces, but few of us address: eliminating the weaknesses in our running form. Injury and disease will attack us at our weakest point, and for us that means that point in our stride at which we are out of alignment and wind up putting more pressure on a place in our bodies than that point was designed to withstand. If learning a new "form" of running means I can stay in alignment and balance more of the time—even when I'm so fatigued I feel like I can barely stand up, much less run—then I will reduce my chance of injury by a huge degree.

You can learn more about ChiRunning at chirunning.com. There are also seminars periodically offered in most regions of the country.

The best way to deal with injuries is to avoid them in the first place.

*What distinguishes those
of us at the starting line from
those of us on the couch is that
we learn through running to
take what the days gives us, what
our body will allow us and
what our will can tolerate.*

JOHN BINGHAM

CHAPTER 8

Running Shoes

ONE OF THE THINGS I love about running is it is such an accessible sport. Think about golf. You need a set of golf clubs. You need golf balls. You need a golf course. Skiing is worse. You need snow. You need a mountain.

You don't need any of that in order to run. In the time it takes you to throw on a pair of shorts and lace up your shoes, you are out the door and into your workout.

Tennis, biking, swimming, working out at a gym—any sport you can think of—requires more equipment, logistics and money than running.

Running is the least expensive sport you can find. The only piece of equipment you need is a good pair of shoes. How long your shoes will last depends on your physical stature and your gait.

Every runner should have two pairs of shoes and alternate them. Part of the reason is that new shoes will have significantly more resilience, and if you switch back and forth between shoes that are newer, and shoes that are somewhat worn, you'll begin to sense when one pair is losing its cushioning and spring. You will begin to know when your older shoes are getting worn and have lost a good deal of their ability to hold your foot in place as you strike the ground. You'll know when they are losing their ability to support the integrity of your feet.

Depending on your weight and how rough you are on your shoes, a good pair will last you 300 to 500 miles. If you run 10 miles per week, that's one pair per year. If you run 20 miles per week and weigh 175 pounds or more, you

How Often Should You Replace Running Shoes?

When running shoes lose their spring and their cushioning, when you can feel the pizzazz fading from them, you should replace them. Worn out running shoes will not protect your feet, ankles and joints as well as a newer pair.

When your shoes start to lose their effectiveness depends on how you use them. There are too many factors to know how many miles, or weeks or months of wear are in an individual runner's shoes.

As a guideline, we've found that lighter runners who weigh 100 pounds or less, and who are not running high mileage, fewer than 15 miles per week, might be able to go up to nine months, perhaps 500 miles, before needing a new pair. Meanwhile, a 200-pound runner who is running 25–50 miles per week might need a new pair every couple months, after 250–300 miles or so.

It's important to remember that a quality pair of running shoes, bought with the advice and recommendation of someone who is knowledgeable and is probably a runner himself or herself, is a necessary investment in terms of your health and your ability to avoid injury and enjoy the sport.

I recommend having two pairs of shoes and alternating between them. If you run in a newer pair and an older pair, then you will continually feel the difference between them, and you'll develop a sense of how old your shoes are when they become too old.

might need three pairs in a year. In any case, it's worth it to buy quality shoes, and the right shoes for you.

◆ ◆ ◆

DETERMINING YOUR FOOT TYPE AND GAIT

UNDERSTANDING PRONATION

The most important concept about the biomechanics of running is pronation. "Pronate" comes from the word "prone," meaning, essentially, "flat." Anything in the prone position is lying flat. When you run, and your foot strikes the ground, it is not in a prone position. In a normal stride, the outside of the foot hits the ground first, beginning with your heel. Look at almost any pair of worn running shoes and you will see more wear on the outside of the heel than the inside.

When the outside of the heel first strikes the ground, there isn't much weight on it. But as you stride forward, all your body weight comes crashing down on your foot, so to speak, and over time, the human body found the most efficient way to deal with it. You might think it would be best if you landed on the middle of your foot and the force of all your weight was distributed from there. But that would create thundering steps like those of a cartoon giant, and since you would be landing in such a solid, stationary position, it would take too much energy to push off and create the next stride.

What actually happens is much better. As your weight comes forward your foot rolls inward, from the outside of the foot to the inside, becoming momentarily flat. In other words, it pronates. In the final phase of your stride, most of your weight is on the inside of your foot and then you push off into your next step. It's a piece of design genius and it accounts for the fact that in the long run, 50 or even 100 miles, humans are the greatest long-distance runners of any animal on the planet.

It's easy to see how "overpronating," i.e., rolling too far inward, or "underpronating," which is also known as "supinating," and means not rolling inward enough, could wreak havoc with your stride and lead to all kinds of injuries. Some runners are fortunate. The way they pronate in their strides is perfect. But most of us fall at least slightly into one category or the other—we pronate a little too much or too little. And, of course, for some of us the imperfection is not slight. We under- or overpronate by a big margin.

ASSESSING YOUR FEET

The first clue to understanding whether you over- or underpronate, or whether your biomechanics are neutral, is to learn what kind of feet you have.

People with flat feet tend to overpronate; there is not enough arch to prevent the natural inward rolling motion of the foot from going too far. Like a bridge that slopes downward, everything rolls downhill.

People with high arches tend to underpronate; the arch is so pronounced it prevents the foot from rolling inward. Like a bridge that slopes upward, it's hard to get across.

You probably already have a sense of what kind of feet you have, but to get a visual reading you can look at your footprint. The classic way is to step barefoot onto a stack of wet newspapers or a brown paper bag, leaving an impression. If the line down the inside of your foot, from the tip of your big toe to your heel is fairly straight, you have flat feet (likelihood of overpronating).

If the line curves significantly inward, leaving an impression that is approximately four inches or more narrower in the middle of your foot than at the top, you have a high arch (likelihood of underpronating).

If the line curves inward but not significantly, less than four inches, and the impression at the middle of your foot is narrower than at the top, but by less than half, your arch is the right height. This doesn't necessarily mean you are not an over- or underpronater. There are other checks you will need to do, but it's a step in the right direction, so to speak.

Another way you can check your pronation proclivity is to study your bare footprint the next time you happen to see it. It might be stepping out of the shower onto a freshly washed bath mat, walking barefoot on a pool deck, or on a recently vacuumed carpet. The next time you are at the beach, walk in wet sand and compare your print to those of other people around you. You'll see all different kinds and get a sense of how extreme or average yours is.

◆ ◆ ◆

HOW TO BUY RUNNING SHOES

GO TO AN INDEPENDENT, SPECIALTY RUNNING SHOE STORE

Stay away from the chain athletic shoe stores, the big sporting goods stores and department stores. Here's why:

- At specialty running stores you'll be buying your shoes from other runners. They understand the sport because they participate in it.
- Company representatives visit specialty stores and spend time educating the employees on the intricacies of their shoes.
- A specialty store sells only running shoes. Employees at chain stores also allegedly know about basketball shoes, cross-trainers, soccer shoes, football cleats, etc. The likelihood that you'll find someone there with a deep understanding of running shoes is slim.
- Matching a runner's foot and gait to the best possible shoe is an art that takes practice. Specialty store personnel get plenty of it.
- Many specialty stores have treadmills you can try out your shoes on, or places outside where employees will watch you run, assessing your needs.

CHECK YOUR SIZE

Don't assume that the size of your foot doesn't change. Many runners new to the sport are wearing shoes that are too short. If you are over 40 or have been pregnant, chances are your feet have become larger over the years. With time, arches tend to flatten and feet become longer. Sometimes that size you have always purchased and been comfortable in has slowly been getting tighter without your noticing. So get your feet measured periodically, and measure both feet because they are not always identical.

Evaluate the size of your current shoes by standing and raising your heels, one at a time, about ½ inch off the floor. Have someone push the end of your shoe in toward your toes. Have them push at several points but begin with your longest toe. If the toe is less than ½ inch from the end of your shoe, then your shoes are too short.

Also, know that brands differ in size. Until you are absolutely certain what size you wear in a particular brand, don't buy your shoes without trying them on. Even if you are certain of your size, our feet change over time, usually growing larger, so at least periodically try on a pair of shoes that are different from your customary size.

BRING AN OLD PAIR WITH YOU

Your old running shoes tell the story of your gait. You have imprinted it there thousands of times, and that's a lot of valuable information. Bring a pair with you and your shoe seller will be able to read what happens when your foot strikes the ground.

On Running Barefoot

There is a small but highly publicized mini-movement within the latest running boom that promotes the idea that we should all run barefoot. The thinking is that if we run without shoes, we'll be able to develop perfect biomechanics and thus become immune from running injuries. Indeed, barefoot running proponents feel that running shoes distort a perfectly natural running form and are therefore the cause of most running injuries.

But if you have ever pulled a small stone, a piece of glass, a thumbtack or worse out of the sole of your running shoe, you understand the common sense that flies in the face of this theory.

Running barefoot is not a good idea for the vast majority of runners. For all but a tiny percentage, the hazards will overwhelmingly outweigh the far-off, theoretical benefits. If you have a perfectionist's mindset, if you typically take the elitist's path, if you have great legs and feet and you feel compelled to give barefoot running a shot, I'll advise you to be clear about the benefits you think you can achieve by taking this course, I'll caution you to be careful and I'll wish you luck.

Is there sound science behind the barefoot running idea? To be fair, I believe there is some, but not a preponderance. Yes, there was a time, thousands of years ago, when Homo sapiens all ran barefoot and were very good at it. But the surfaces they were running on were different than what we have today, and we have moved up the evolutionary chain quite a bit since then. We live indoors, we work in offices, we wear professional dress and there are some pretty good reasons why businesses, even in beach towns, hang signs that say, "No shoes, no service."

Meanwhile, the development of running shoes has helped make running the number one participant sport in the world. Without running shoes there wouldn't be any marathons outside the Olympics, nor would you see runners on the streets of every town in America as well other nations around the globe. When you factor in the improved health enjoyed by tens of millions of runners worldwide, and the increased longevity, running shoes are among the great inventions of the 20th century. (I'm not aware of anyone running the numbers, so to speak, but if you calculated the financial savings in terms of reduced health care costs, running shoes might also be among the greatest cost-saving inventions as well.)

Finally, the fine book, "Born to Run," by Christopher McDougall, which introduced us to the Tarahumara tribe of native North Americans who live in the Mexican desert and are some of the world's greatest long-distance runners, has been used as a touchstone by the barefoot running proponents. The Tarahumara are great, natural runners whose habits and style of running hark back thousands of years, and they are hugely successful as runners so we should do everything we can to emulate them.

Perhaps. That said, even the Tarahumara have footwear—sandal-like shoes made from tire treads.

It's unlikely that the first humans who began strapping things to the bottoms of their feet to make ambulating more comfortable and effective were following an incorrect evolutionary impulse. I'm pretty sure that if Og the Caveman had Nikes or Sauconys available to him, he'd have worn them and he'd have caught and killed more mastodons or elk or whatever he was pursuing.

THE RIGHT PAIR FOR YOUR FEET

Shoes are divided into three basic categories: ***Motion Controlled, Cushioned*** and ***Stability.***

Motion Control Shoes

These shoes are built to prevent the feet of runners who overpronate from rolling in too far. They have a straight shape and provide more support than any other shoe design. They are the most rigid and control-oriented shoes. If you have flat feet, these are probably the shoes in which you will feel and perform best.

Cushioned Shoes

These shoes have a curved shape designed to encourage the foot of a runner who underprontates to roll inward more than it naturally does. They have the softest midsole and the least medial support of any kind of shoe. If you have high arches, these are probably the shoes in which you will feel and perform best.

Stability Shoes

These shoes are designed to provide runners with normal arches who pronate normally a neutral balance of cushioning, medial support and durability.

◆ ◆ ◆

HOW TO LACE RUNNING SHOES

The two guidelines for lacing running shoes are to create a snug fit so your shoes do not slip, which will lead to rubbing and friction; and at the same time don't lace them so tightly that they limit circulation or constrict nerves.

Several nerves run across the top of the foot and it's easy to squeeze them by lacing your shoes too tightly. Laces that are too tight limit blood flow to these nerves, which causes tingling or numbness. The tricky situation is that these nerves can be compressed even though your shoes don't feel too tight. When runners feel their toes or the front part of the foot going tingly or numb, they often suspect much more complicated troubles than shoes that are too tightly laced.

Another common problem connected to lacing is tendonitis on top of the foot. Like the nerves, the tendons on top of the foot are close to the surface and tight laces can rub against them causing inflammation, or tendonitis, and it can be painful.

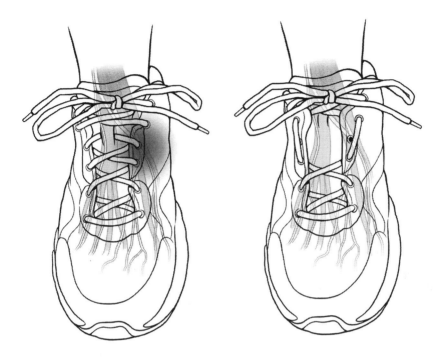

AN ALTERNATE LACING PATTERN CAN EASE THE PRESSURE ON SENSITIVE NERVES AND TENDONS LOCATED ON THE TOP OF THE FOOT.

The solution in either situation is to loosen the laces, but loosening all the laces can lead to your shoes slipping in other places.

The way to loosen your laces only in that spot is to "skiplace" your shoes, meaning don't thread your laces through the eyehole in the particular spot where you are experiencing the tightness. Usually, the eyehole you'll skip will be the second or the third down from the top of the shoe depending on the configuration of eyeholes in your type of shoe. You may want to experiment with different lacing patterns that include skipping the affected area but still keep your shoes significantly snug.

You can quickly remedy the situation with a trip to your specialty running shoe store. The people there have seen this problem many times before and they can show you lacing patterns that will eliminate it; and once you are aware of it, they can recommend shoes that will help you avoid it in the first place.

CARING FOR YOUR RUNNING SHOES

Here are tips for getting the most out of your shoes.

- Get a second pair and alternate. If you run several times a week, this will allow them sufficient time to dry and for the cushioning material to completely rebound.
- Untie the laces before taking them off, rather than stepping on the heels.
- Dry them slowly using cool temperatures. Don't dry them near a very hot source, such as on a radiator. This will break down and crack the rubber and other materials.
- If they get dirty, you can throw them in the washing machine, but not the dryer.
- Replacing your shoes after 300-400 miles is the conventional wisdom. Depending on your weight and the degree to which you stress your shoes, you might need new shoes sooner than this, or later. You can check by taking them into your specialty running shoe store and trying a new shoe on one foot while wearing your old shoe on the other. How stark is the difference? How do your feet and legs feel in each shoe?

◆ ◆ ◆

RECYCLING YOUR SHOES

Running shoes are one of the most recyclable commodities you can buy. Nike will tear them apart and reuse the three main components in a variety of ways. After fewer than 500 miles, your shoes may not be ideal to run in, but they will have plenty of life to offer someone who simply needs something to wear on his or her feet. Here are recycling sources to explore.

- *soles4souls.org* was founded to help victims of Hurricanes Rita and Katrina and the Asian Tsunami of 2004 and donates gently worn shoes to people in need. Visit the site to find a convenient drop-off location (quite possibly your running shoe store).
- *shoe4africa.org* has been sending running shoes to Kenya to prevent disease and encourage participation in the sport since 1995. They're also building a hospital. Visit the site for instructions on how you can send shoes with 100 miles of wear left in them directly to Kenya.
- *nikereuseashoe.com* breaks shoes into three parts for reuse. Some pieces become tracks, tennis courts or other athletic surfaces, while others get recycled back into new shoes. Collection points include all Nike stores.

Should You Stretch Before or After a Run?

Many studies differ in their results and advice on this question—one in particular showed more injuries occurring in runners who stretch before they run, but that goes counter to everything we have ever learned. The Pasadena Pacers seem to incur a much lower rate of injury than most groups of runners and I attribute this, in part, to the fact that we stretch and warm up before every run. We take our time, about 15 minutes, and we do a thorough job. We are led as a group by one of a number of our members who understand the principles behind stretching out and warming up slowly. They present the stretches in proper sequence and demonstrate them correctly. It is common sense that if your muscles are warm and at least somewhat lengthened before you begin stressing, they will be more prepared and suffer less damage, so I believe in stretching before the run.

At the same time, many studies have shown that stretching afterward prevents injury. Once the muscles are heated and stressed, and lactic acid has been released into the system, you want to close the system down gradually. I believe this helps the natural healing process. Even for non-athletes, a day's activities stress the body; that's why people who don't exercise at all are still sore at the end of the day. Elite runners would never end their workouts with a sprint to the finish line and then head straight for the showers. Trainers would never take a thoroughbred horse back to the barn after a race without cooling it down first. And after you are done using your computer, when you have eight windows open, you don't simply pull the plug out of the wall. I believe the proper thing after a hard workout is to cool down with some light jogging or walking, and then stretch for ten minutes.

So the answer to the question—stretch before or after?—is, "both."

Running should be a
lifelong activity. Approach
it patiently and intelligently,
and it will reward you
for a long, long time.

MICHAEL SARGENT

CHAPTER 9

Stretching &
Strengthening Exercises

YOUR STRETCHING AND STRENGTHENING program is only as good as the likelihood that you will use it. You can have a color, glossy chart on your wall showing how to do 87 exercises, with photos of the world's fittest, most beautiful people demonstrating them, but if you don't do them, all is for naught.

Most runners would rather spend their time running than doing stretching and strengthening exercises. We're not into equipment. The gym is not our idea of a good time. We don't like workouts that support our running. We just want to run.

Time is scarce. If you're training for a particular race, or if you are ambitious about getting faster, working out on a mat can seem like wasted time. *How can I achieve my running goals if I am practicing bending over and touching my toes?* I've heard that complaint more than once.

In the long run—no pun intended—that's faulty thinking. These supportive workouts actually save time and create more running opportunities, as well as make you a better runner. Let's do the math. If you work out three times a week, that's about 150 workouts per year. If you devote one quarter of one workout per week to stretching and strengthening exercises, measured in total time, that comes to about 12 full running workouts per year. That seems like a lot.

But if you get injured and can't run for six weeks, you miss 18 workouts, which is 50% more than if you had dedicated a small amount of time to stretching and strengthening. But it gets worse. Missing all those workouts consecutively destroys your fitness. You will have to train for months to get back to the level you had achieved. If you had plans to run a race, they go down the drain as well.

My hope is to persuade you to build regular stretching and strengthening sessions into your workout program. This chapter contains more than 40 stretches, exercises and plyometrics. Mix and match to customize your workout to your injuries and to strengthen all the areas key to runners.

But the best feature of many of these exercises is something you probably have never heard of before. You'll find most of these exercises to be closed chained exercises, meaning when you do them the energy moves in a closed kinetic system. A pushup is a closed chain exercise because the energy you send into the ground comes back in the form of resistance. An example of an open chain would be putting a weight on the end of your foot and swinging it through the air; the energy leaves and does not return.

The advantage of closed chain exercises is they train your central nervous system to maintain the integrity of your gait even when you are running through fatigue. The majority of injuries occur when we run tired and our stride falls off kilter, creating more stress on one area of the body than it can handle. These exercises tune your nervous system to fire your muscles rapidly in the proper sequence, and that holds your body in line. Several of these exercises will help you improve your balance, also boosting your ability to hold your body in line, not to mention they are great strengtheners.

In addition to exercises and stretches, I have added a number of plyometric exercises, or "plyos." Plyos are a training technique designed to increase muscular strength and power. They condition the body by providing individual muscles with resistance for brief periods of time. They rapidly stretch and then shorten a muscle with motions such as hopping and jumping. This brief, intense and repetitive working of the muscle makes it stronger and better able to "explode" when it's called upon for short bursts of movement, such as a runner's stride.

A word of caution about plyos: You should build up a base of running strength before taking on plyometrics. A good threshold for this base is 25 to 35 miles of running per week for a period of six weeks, plus three weeks of performing several of the basic exercises listed in this section on a daily basis. While plyos are a great way to condition your body to avoid injury, taking on plyos before your body is ready risks injury.

If we can train ourselves to keep our running form intact throughout our workouts, we can avoid most of the injuries we now face.

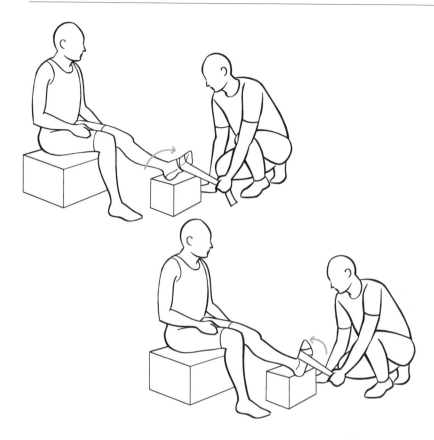

SHIN STRENGTHENING 1

❶ Sit in a low chair or on a stool and extend your left leg outward. It helps to rest your ankle on a couple of yoga blocks or a stool about 12 inches off the ground with your foot hanging over the edge, but you can do this exercise resting your heel on the ground.

❷ Wrap a Thera-Band around the top of your foot and tie it to a bedpost or some stationary object just a couple inches above the ground and 12 inches or fewer forward of your foot; better yet, have a buddy hold the band in this position. Make sure the band is tight enough to provide resistance but not so tight as to prevent you from doing 12 reps with perfect form.

❸ With the band providing resistance, and your left leg, ankle and heel stationary, draw the top of your left foot up and toward your right shoulder as far as you can; then push down and out extending your left big toe as far from your right shoulder as you can.

❹ Do 12 reps and then reverse feet.

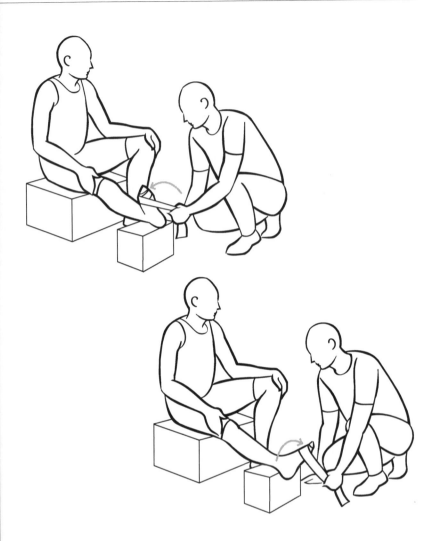

SHIN STRENGTHENING 2

❶ Set yourself up exactly the same as you did for "Shin Strengthening 1" with your left leg extended and a Thera-Band limiting the movement of your left foot.

❷ This time, draw your left foot up and out, toward the outside of your left shoulder.

❸ Then push it down and in, as far from your left shoulder as you can.

❹ Do 12 repeats if you can, as long as you maintain perfect form.

❺ Switch legs and repeat.

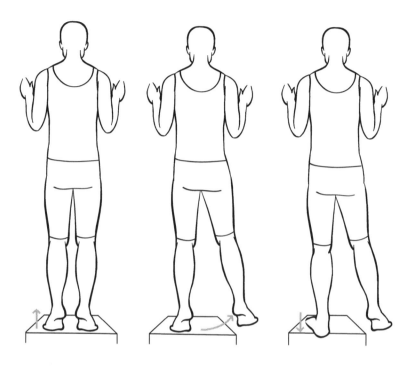

HEAVY LOAD ECCENTRIC CONTRACTION

This is a great exercise for strengthening and stretching an injured leg or ankle (for instance the Achilles tendon and/or the other tendons that support the ankle). Make sure you are sufficiently recovered from the injury so that your affected leg can support your full body weight. The focus of this exercise is on completing the healing process and strengthening the injured leg, ankle and foot to minimize the chances of re-injuring it.

❶ Stand on a step or a stool and let your heels hang off the edge.

❷ With your feet just a few inches apart, transfer all your weight to your injured leg.

❸ Now rise up on your injured leg, flexing and extending the foot on that side as far as you can.

❹ Hold for a moment at the top and then slowly lower down. You should take at least three times longer coming down as going up.

❺ Work on this until you can do 12 repeats with the recovering leg.

EXERCISES

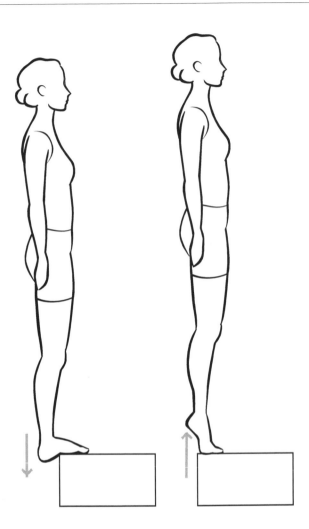

ACHILLES PRESS

❶ Stand on a step or a stool with both heels hanging off the edge.

❷ With your feet just a couple inches apart, lower your heels as far as you can and then raise up on your toes.

❸ Hold for a moment and lower slowly back down.

❹ Work up to three sets of 15.

For stability, touch a wall or banister in front of you or to one side. To make the exercise easier, lean forward and steady yourself on a wall, then raise up. Great for stretching and strengthening calf muscles and Achilles tendon.

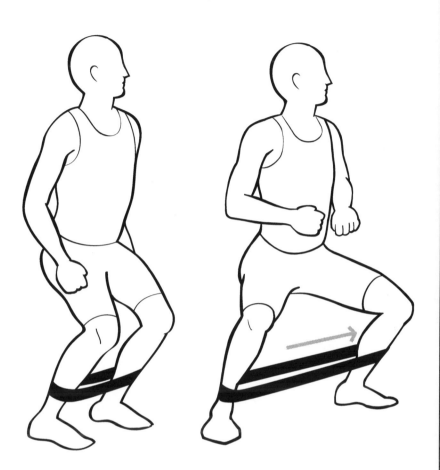

THERA-BAND CRAB WALK

❶ With a Thera-Band around your ankles, lower into a squat. The lower you can go, the better the workout. Keep your back straight; don't lean forward.

❷ With your right foot stationary, take a wide step to the left. The band will provide resistance.

❸ Take three to four lateral steps, about 15 feet, and then return; that's one repeat.

❹ Do ten repeats.

Great for your IT band, quadriceps and ankles. The wider you step, the tougher the workout.

EXERCISES

EXERCISES

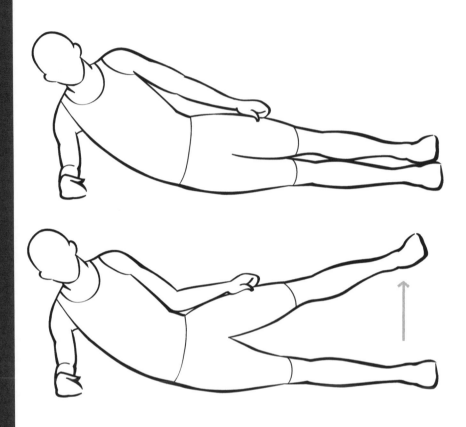

SIDE-LYING HIP ABDUCTION

❶ Lie on your left side propping yourself up with your left arm.

❷ Now raise your right leg (your top leg) as far as you can, and hold for one second, then slowly lower down. Keep both legs straight.

❸ Reverse sides. Do sets of 15.

Great for your groin muscles, hip flexors and IT band.

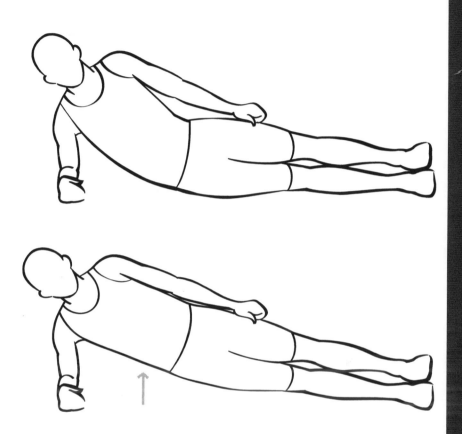

LYING SIDE PLANK

❶ Lie on your left side propping yourself up with your left arm.

❷ Raise your left hip off the floor so your body is straight, your weight on your left forearm. Hold for 30 seconds.

❸ Raise your right arm pointing straight overhead to add difficulty.

❹ Reverse sides.

Great for your abdominals and core, and hip flexors.

EXERCISES

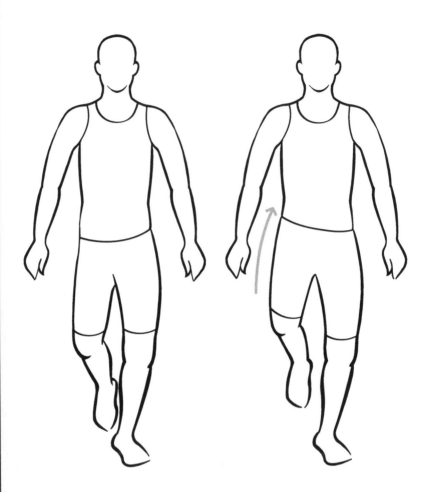

HIP HIKE

❶ With your left foot flat on the floor, raise your right foot off the ground.

❷ Then keeping your left foot flat against the ground, hike your right hip up, hold briefly and then return.

❸ Do 50 per day on both sides in any combination.

To add difficulty, put the end of a Thera-Band underneath your left foot and hold the other end taut in your right hand. The band will provide resistance as you move your hip upward.

This strengthens your gluteus maximus muscles and helps prevents your hips from swinging out of alignment as you run, particularly near the end of a run when you may be fatigued. This is a great exercise for new runners in particular.

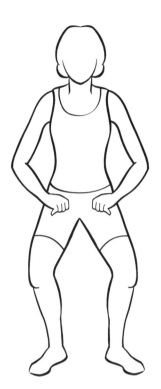
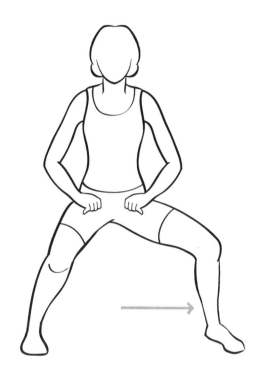

SUMO WALK

❶ With your feet shoulder width apart, squat as deeply as you can without your knees exceeding 45 degrees.

❷ Step laterally to the left taking three to four wide steps until you cover a distance of about 15 feet.

❸ Reverse and go back the other way.

❹ Do 20 passes, ten in each direction.

This exercise is the same as the "Crab Walk," except it's done without the Thera-Band, making it an easier alternative.

EXERCISES

EXERCISES

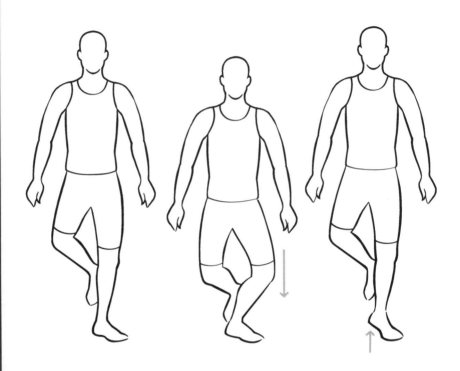

ONE LEGGED PLIÉ

❶ Stand with your feet pointed out 30–45 degrees.

❷ Raise your left foot off the ground so you are standing on your right.

❸ Stabilize yourself and then squat down about 30% of your maximum.

❹ Stand back up into a toe raise as high as you can go.

❺ Lower back down to standing. Stay as centered as you can, avoiding the tendency to tip to the right.

❻ Work up to three sets of 12 with each leg.

This exercise strengthens the inside of your thigh, your calf and the arch of your foot, and it helps prevent kneecap tracking problems that cause pain on the inside of your knee, which is common for new runners.

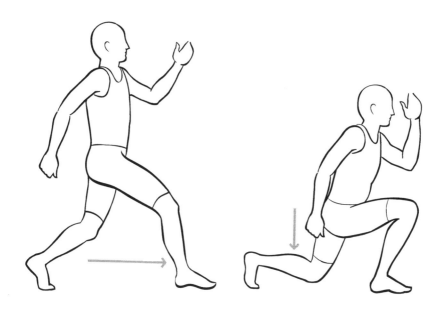

WALKING LUNGE

❶ Begin by taking a giant step forward with your right foot.

❷ As you hold this lunge, lower your left (back) knee to within 2 to 4 inches of the ground.

❸ Then rise up and step forward repeating the lunge with your left foot.

As you do these lunges maintain good runner's form by exaggerating your arm movements as well as your legs. As you step forward, raise your opposite arm with your elbow pointing forward, your fingers pointing up and your bicep parallel with the ground. Practicing this strong, classic runner's pose will help you integrate good form into your running posture, which is a great hedge against injury.

EXERCISES

EXERCISES

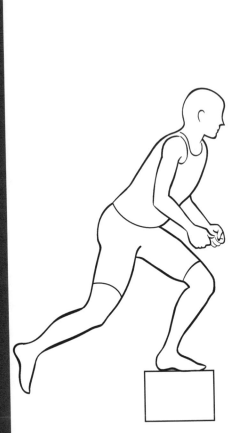 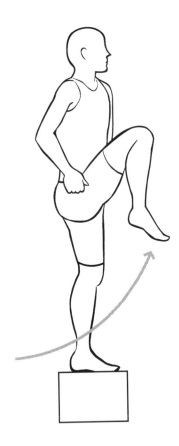

KNEE DRIVE

❶ Stand on a stool or a step and balance on your left foot.

❷ Once you're stable, squat so your left knee comes to a 45-degree angle, your right toes touching the ground for only a moment.

❸ Then rise up as forcefully as you can, fully extending your left leg. Drive your right knee up as high and as quickly as you can, all the way to your chest if possible.

❹ Do two sets of ten with each leg.

This exercise is terrific for strengthening your quadriceps, which will improve your power and stamina as you run.

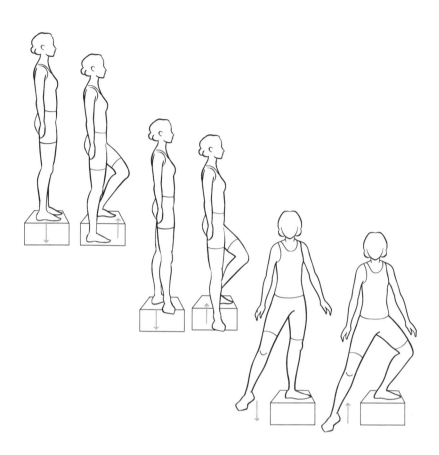

THREE WAY STEP DOWN

❶ Stand on a stool or a step. If you are using a step face sideways so you can drop one foot lower than floor height keeping it alongside the other foot.

❷ Stand on your left foot facing forward, stabilize, and then squat as low as you can, suspending your right foot.

❸ Then lower your right foot as far as it can go without touching the ground.

❹ Work up to sets of 15 on each leg.

For a variation, repeat the exercise with your right foot turned outward, facing to the right, perpendicular to your left leg.

Pose 1

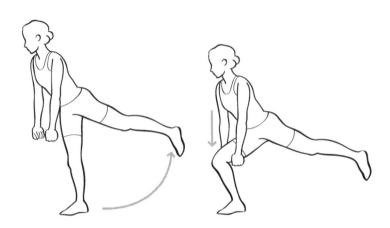

FOUR WAY CROSS

Pose 1: Extend your raised leg backward as far as you can while keeping it straight, and then do the knee bends.

Pose 2: Extend the raised leg out to the side.

Pose 3: Extend your raised foot forward as far as you can, straightening your leg and keeping it as straight as possible.

Pose 4: Extend the raised leg across the midline of your body behind you, so the raised foot is on the opposite side, outside the foot you're standing on.

❶ Sink all your weight into your right foot, raise your left foot and stabilize.

❷ Position your left leg in one of the four poses above.

❸ Now do a knee bend lowering down as far as you can go while maintaining your balance.

❹ Rise up and repeat through the other poses.

Pose 2

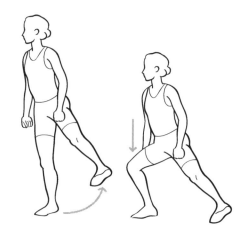

Pose 3

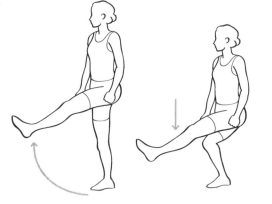

Pose 4

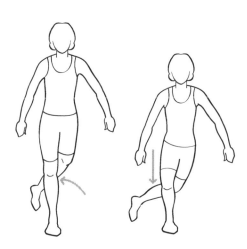

EXERCISES

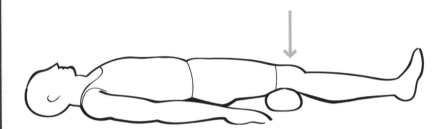

SUPINE QUAD PRESS

❶ Lie down on the floor with a pillow beneath your knees.

❷ Push your knees down into the floor as hard as you can and hold for ten
seconds.

❸ Do two sets of 12.

The thicker and spongier the pillow, the greater the resistance and the harder
this exercise will work your quads and gluteals.

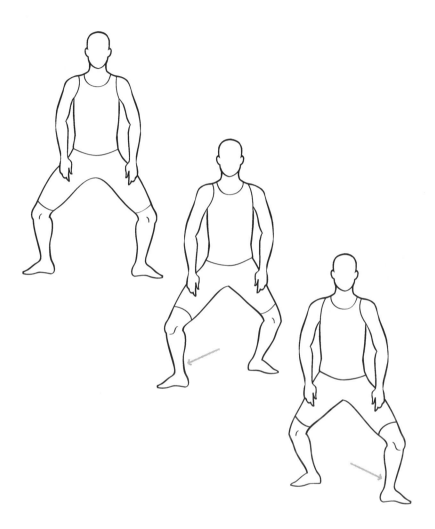

GROUCHO

❶ Stand up straight and go into a deep squat, knees bent just less than a 90-degree angle and thighs at about a 45-degree angle to the floor.

❷ Turn your feet outward as far as you can, so that they are pointing at the walls to either side, and walk forward in this position for several strides, about 15 feet.

❸ Turn around and return. Do 12 repeats.

EXERCISES

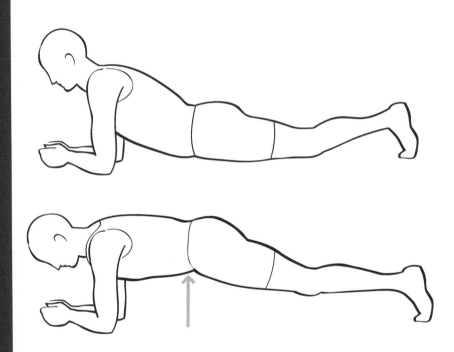

PRONE PLANK

❶ From a hands and knees position on the ground, rise up supporting yourself on your forearms with your elbows bent at 90 degrees and directly beneath your shoulders.

❷ Extend your legs behind you in a pushup position with only your toes touching the ground.

❸ Hold yourself in Prone Plank for 30 seconds or as long as you can. Work up to one minute.

❹ Do three sets.

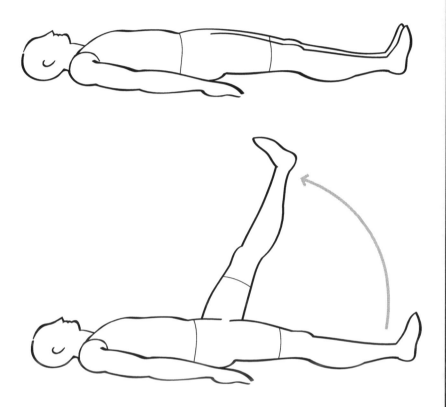

SINGLE STRAIGHT LEG RAISE

❶ Lying flat on the ground, hands at your sides, raise one leg to a 45-degree angle and hold it there for a count of ten.

❷ Then lower it down and repeat. Do ten repeats on each side.

This exercise works your core including your psoas muscles, which are among the chief supporting muscles for runners.

EXERCISES

EXERCISES

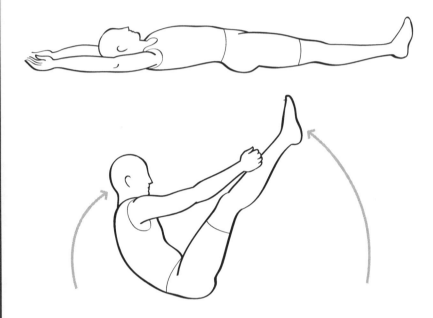

V-SIT

❶ Lie down with your arms stretched overhead

❷ Then sit up into a "V" position, simultaneously raising your legs to about a 45-degree angle to the floor. Reach with your fingertips and touch your toes if you can. If not, reach for a point on your leg closer to your knees.

❸ Hold at the top for a moment and then lie back down.

❹ Do as many as you can, working up to two sets of ten.

This is an intense exercise that strengthens all the core muscles.

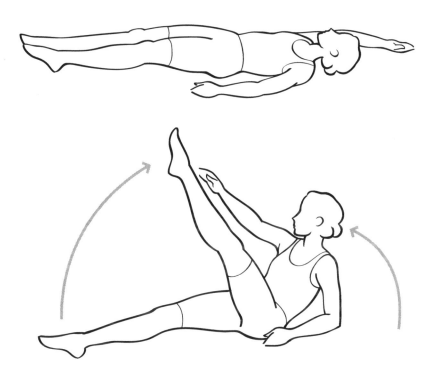

ONE LEG V-SIT

❶ Lie down with your right arm stretched overhead and your left arm at your side.

❷ Sit up and raise your left leg to a 45-degree angle without bending your leg and reach across your body with your right hand and, if you can, touch your left toes.

❸ Keep your left leg as straight as possible.

❹ Reverse sides. Do ten repeats and two sets.

EXERCISES

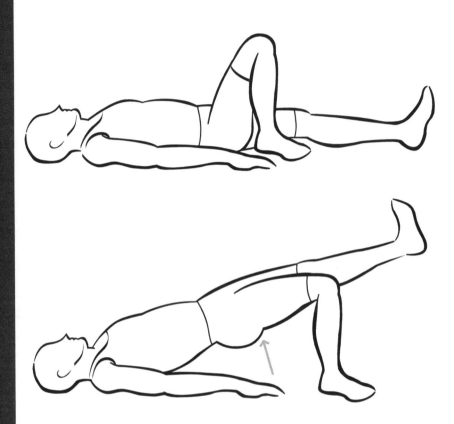

BUTT PRESS

❶ Lie on your back with your left leg straight out and your right leg bent, your foot flat on the floor.

❷ With your hands at your sides, push down into the ground with your right foot and raise your butt and your left leg off the floor. Keep your left leg straight as you hold this position for 20 seconds. Breathe into this stretch.

❸ Reverse legs. Work up to two sets of ten.

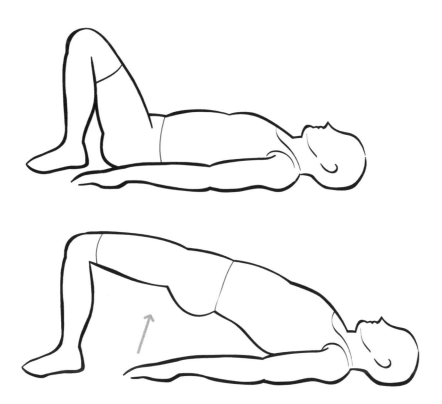

BRIDGING

❶ Lie on your back with both feet flat on the floor, your heels just outside and slightly beneath your hips.

❷ With your hands at your sides, press down into your feet and raise your butt as high off the ground as you can, and hold. As you hold for ten seconds, no part of your body from beneath your shoulders to your heels is touching the ground.

❸ Do two sets of ten repeats.

EXERCISES

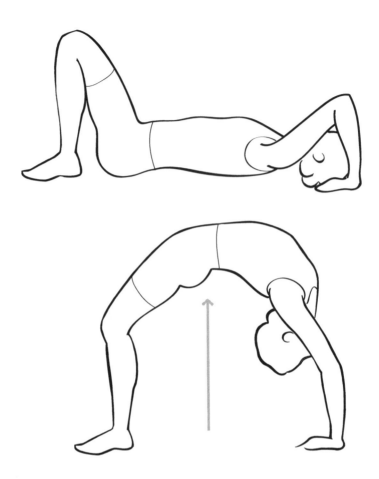

WRESTLER'S BRIDGE

❶ Lie on your back with your feet flat on the ground, your heels just outside and slightly lower than your hips.

❷ Place your hands next to your ears with your fingers pointing toward your feet, and press down with both your hands and feet.

❸ Extend your arms and your legs so your elbows and knees are as straight as possible, your back arched, your pelvis raised as high as possible.

❹ Hold this position for a count of ten and then lower down carefully.

❺ Work up to two sets of ten repeats.

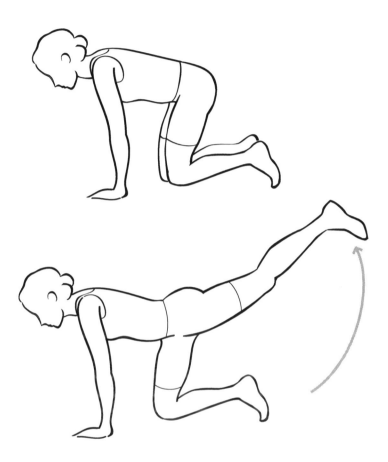

DONKEY KICKS

❶ Kneel on all fours in the "table" position, your hands beneath your shoulders.

❷ Pick up your left leg and extend it backwards, straightening your knee and raising your foot as high behind you as you can.

❸ Hold there a moment and then bring your left leg forcefully forward touching your left knee to your chest.

❹ Kick your leg backward again as far as you can, and bring your knee forward again to your chest.

❺ Do ten repeats and then switch legs. Work up to two sets.

EXERCISES

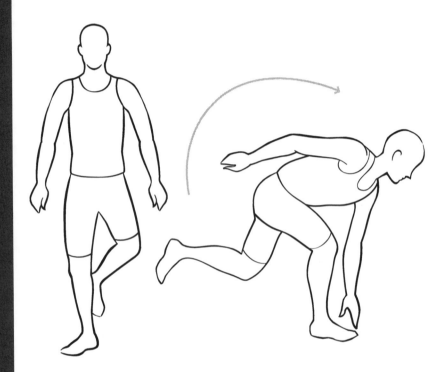

BUTT BLASTER

❶ Stand on your right leg and bending your right knee and leaning forward, use your left hand to touch the outside of your right foot.

❷ Rise up to a standing position on your right leg without your left foot touching the ground.

❸ Do ten repeats and switch legs. Work up to three sets.

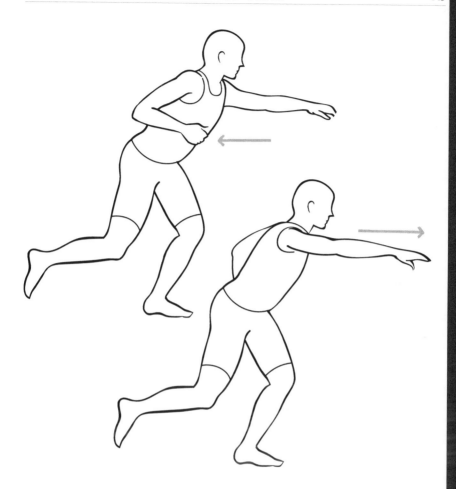

FIRE BUCKETS

❶ Stand on your right leg, your left leg raised a few inches, and lower yourself down, bending slightly forward. Your right knee should make about a 45-degree angle.

❷ Stabilize yourself and then reach forward with your right hand as far as you can, as if you were grabbing a bucket.

❸ Pull your right hand back and then reach forward with your left hand. Alternate hands to a count of 20.

❹ Switch legs. Work up to three sets.

This exercise is great for stabilizing your subtle hip muscles, which will improve your posture as you run.

EXERCISES

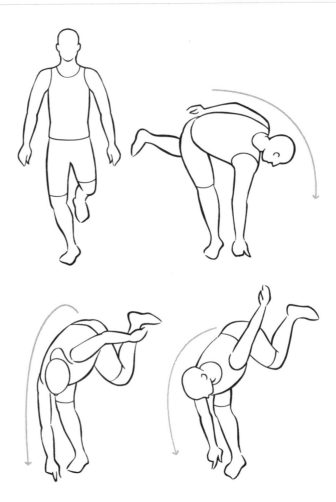

THREE POINT TOUCH

❶ Stand on the right leg, and bend the right knee.

❷ Using your right hand, reach to the inside of the right heel taking your left leg up, and touching about two inches from the right heel while maintaining balance without touching the other foot to the ground. Switch legs and then do other side.

❸ Now standing at the starting position and bending your right knee, reach to two inches in front of the toe with your right hand. Do other side.

❹ Reach to about two inches to the outside of the right heel. Do other side.

❺ Do two sets of 12 repetitions for each exercise.

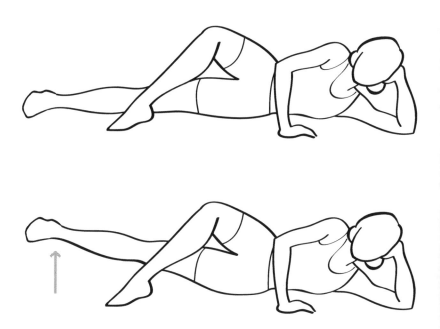

HIP ADDUCTOR

❶ Lie on your left side leaning on your left elbow, your head resting in your left hand.

❷ Cross your right leg over your left knee with your right foot flat on the ground.

❸ Now raise your left leg as high as you can, keeping it straight, and hold for a moment before lowering it back down.

❹ Switch legs. Do two sets of ten repeats.

This exercise works the muscles on the inside of the thigh including the adductor, or groin muscles.

EXERCISES

PLYOMETRICS

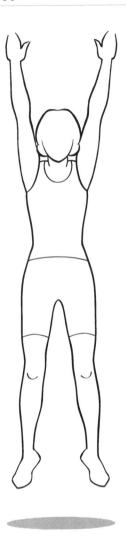
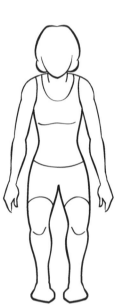

ROCKET JUMPS

❶ From a standing position, go into a squat with your quads at about a 45-degree angle to the floor.

❷ Then jump as high as you can, extending your arms straight overhead.

❸ As you come down let your momentum bring you down into a squat before firing straight back up into your next jump.

❹ Work up to three sets of ten.

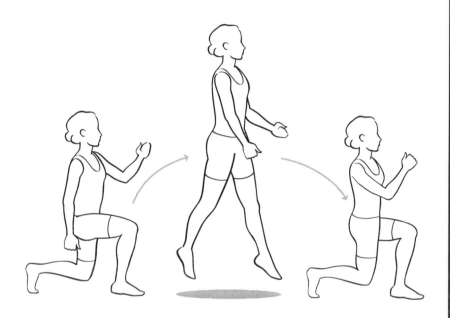

LUNGE SPRING

❶ From a standing position, take a long lunging stride forward with your left leg. Let your right arm come forward with your elbow at a 90-degree angle, your right hand pointed straight up. As you lunge or stride, your opposite arm swings forward. At the front of your lunge both knees will be at 90-degree angles.

❷ Now jump and switch legs so that as you come down you are in the lunge position but with both legs and arms reversed.

❸ Work up to three sets of ten.

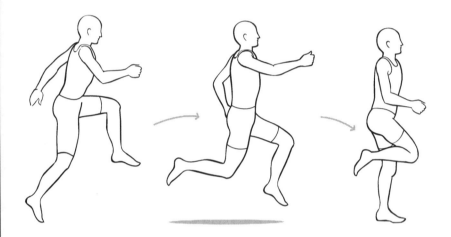

BOUNDING

❶ In this exercise you simply run forward, but exaggerate your steps by extending your knee as high as you can on your forward bound, and also extending your back leg as far as you can.

❷ At the top of your stride, hold each leg for a moment in its fully extended position. Your forward leg should come up so that your knee is in a 90-degree angle, and at the same moment your back leg should be completely straight, your feet fully flexed with your toes off the ground.

❸ Take 15 strides forward, then turn around and repeat.

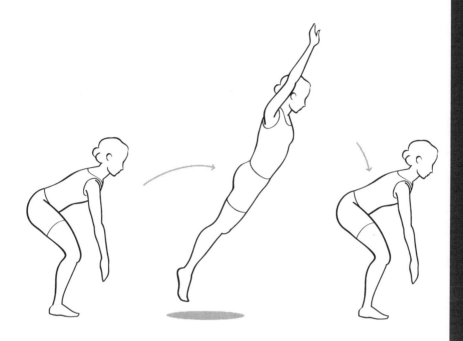

FROG JUMP

❶ From a standing position, go into a full squat with your knees bent at greater than a 90-degree angle, your butt nearly touching the floor.

❷ Jump as high and as far as you can. This is an exaggerated standing broad jump. To aid in momentum, swing your arms backward slightly before you jump and then all the way forward as you go into your jump.

❸ Do ten jumps forward, then turn around and do ten back the other way.

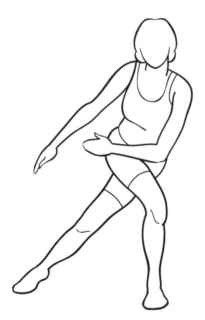 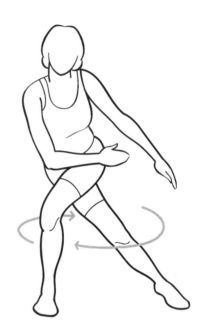

SPEED SKATER

❶ From a standing position, jump forward landing on your left foot. As you jump, cross your right foot behind your left leg and raise it so that your right calf is parallel to the ground. This will tug your right hip back giving it a nice extension and gently pulling you into a speed skater position.

❷ As you jump-stride forward, thrust your opposite arm ahead in good running form.

❸ Hold for a half second when you are fully extended but let your momentum carry you forward from stride to stride.

❹ Do 12 strides forward, then turn around and do 12 back the other way.

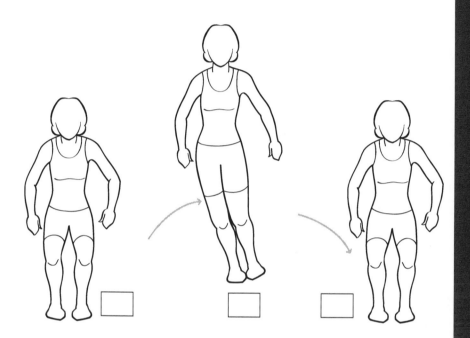

SIDE HURDLE

❶ Stand alongside a small box such as a book box, and jump laterally over the box as high and as far as you can. Jump and land with both feet together.

❷ As you touch down, jump immediately back in the other direction. You don't necessarily need a box to jump over. Any object that does not present an injury risk will suffice, even a workout towel placed on the ground; or you can omit the object and simply jump back and forth.

❸ Work up to three sets of 12 repeats.

PLYOMETRICS

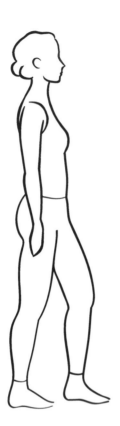
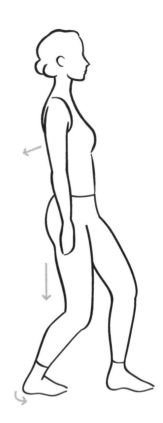

LOWER CALF

❶ From a standing position, step your left leg forward a quarter to a half step.

❷ With your left foot flat on the ground, turn your right (back) heel out slightly, just a few inches, and bend your right (back) leg far enough that your right heel comes off the ground slightly.

❸ Lean backward just until you feel the stretch in the lower portion of your right calf.

❹ Hold for a slow count of ten and breathe into the stretch.

This stretch is also great for your Achilles tendon and the plantar fascia, the tendons and soft tissue in the bottom of your foot.

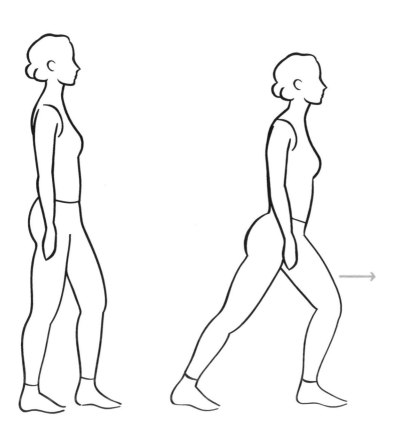

UPPER CALF

❶ From a standing position, take a half step forward with your left leg, straighten the back of the right (back) knee, turn the right heel outward just a few inches and lean forward with most of your weight on your left leg.

❷ Keep your right leg straight so that you feel the stretch in the back of your leg below your knee, in your upper calf.

❸ Hold for a slow count of ten and breathe into the stretch.

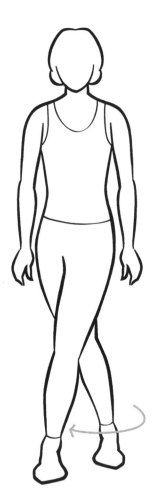
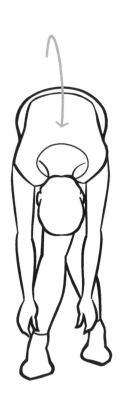

HAMSTRING

❶ From a standing position, cross your right foot over your left so your feet are alongside one another.

❷ Bend forward hinging at the waist and allow the weight of your torso to pull your chest gently toward the tops of your feet and, if you can, folding against your knees. Keep your left (back) leg straight.

❸ Extend gently until you feel a slightly uncomfortable stretch in your hamstring and hold for a slow count of ten. Breathe into the stretch.

❹ Switch legs, crossing your left over your right and then repeat.

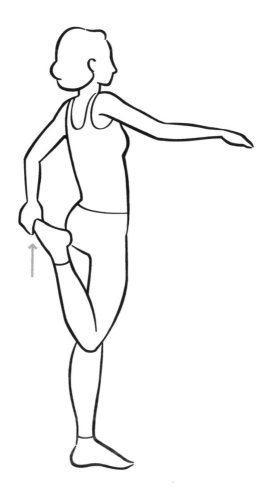

QUAD/SHIN DOUBLE STRETCH

❶ From a standing position, raise your right leg and with your left hand, reach
behind and grab the top of your right foot.

❷ Pull your foot in as close to the left side of your butt as you can so that you
feel a stretch in the front of your right thigh (quadriceps) and the front of your
right calf.

❸ Hold for a slow count of ten and breathe into the stretch. Switch legs
and repeat.

This stretch will work the front calf muscles where shin splints can occur, as well
as the muscles and tendons in the lower calf and ankle.

STRETCHES

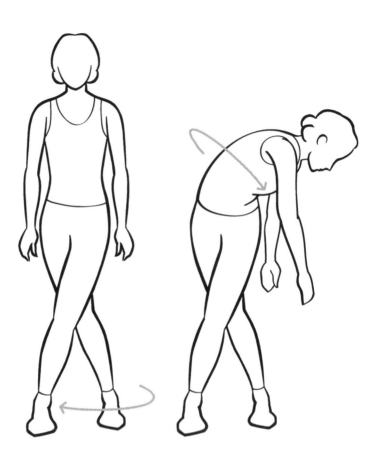

ILLIOTIBIAL BAND

❶ From a standing position, cross your right leg over your left positioning your right foot about 12 inches to the left of your left foot, and with your right heel even with the toes on your left foot.

❷ Now bend at the waist and twist to the right as far as you can, reaching with both hands for the outside of your left foot.

❸ Extend gently until you feel the stretch on the outside of your right leg just below your waist.

❹ Breathe into the stretch and hold for a slow count of ten.

❺ Switch legs and repeat.

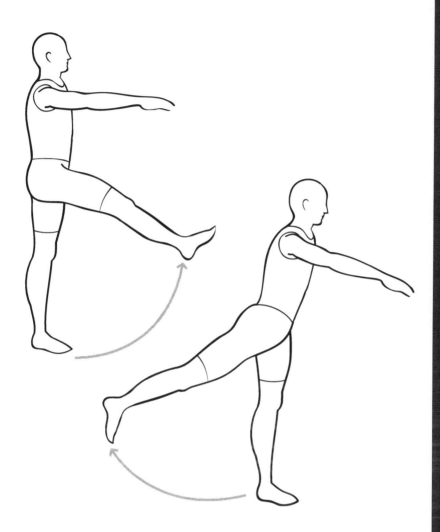

SCISSOR KICK

❶ From a standing position, raise your right foot and swing your right leg backward as far as you can and then forward as far as you can.

❷ As your leg swings backward let your momentum carry it back as far as it can go. You can stretch your arms out to the sides to help you maintain balance. Keeping both legs as straight as possible will increase the stretch in the back of both legs.

❸ Do ten kicks and then switch legs and repeat. Do two sets.

STRETCHES

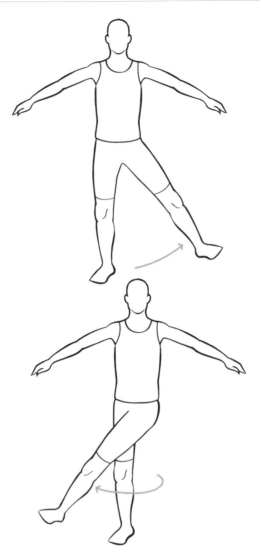

SIDE SCISSORS

❶ From a standing position, kick your right leg to the left, passing it in front of your left leg in a sweeping motion and extending it as far to the left as you can.

❷ Then swing it back the other way, extending it as far out to the right as you can.

❸ Continue kicking across to the left and out to the right for ten repeats.

❹ Switch legs and repeat. Do two sets.

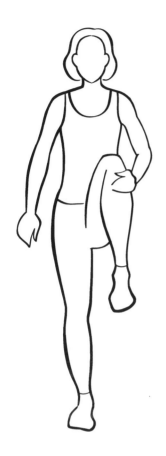 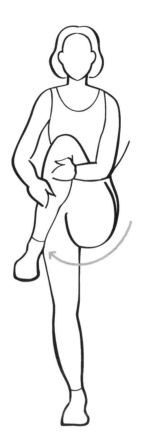

HIP

❶ From a standing position, raise your right leg and with your right hand, pull your knee up.

❷ With your left hand, grab your right ankle or your right leg just above the ankle, stabilize your balance and then use both hands to gently pull your right leg up further and toward your left shoulder.

❸ Extend gently until you feel a good stretch in your right gluteal muscle and the outside of your right hip.

❹ Hold for a slow count of ten, then reverse and repeat the exercise with your left leg.

❺ Do two sets.

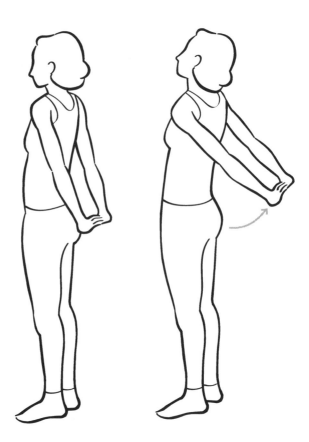

UPPER CHEST

❶ From a standing position, clasp your hands behind your back with your palms facing away from your body.

❷ Straighten your elbows, arch your back and push your hands as far away from your body as you can, while reaching them up as far as they will go. Tighten your abs and level your pelvis, meaning, don't allow it to tip forward. Keep your head erect and slightly back.

❸ Extend your hands up and push them gently away from your body as far as possible until you feel a good stretch in your shoulders, arms and back, as well as the front of your neck, your chest and ribs.

❹ With each exhale, extend the stretch slightly further.

❺ Gently hold for a slow count of ten, shake out your arms and do one more set.

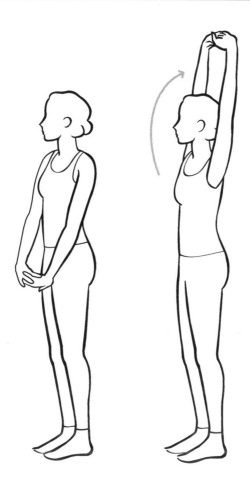

LOWER CHEST

❶ From a standing position, clasp your hands with your palms facing away from your body.

❷ Straighten your elbows, arch your back and push your hands as far away from your body as you can, while reaching them up as far as they will go. Tighten your abs and level your pelvis, meaning, don't allow it to tip forward. Keep your head erect and slightly back.

❸ Push for the sky, reach as far back as possible and hold your head level.

❹ With each exhale, extend the stretch slightly further.

❺ Gently hold for a slow count of ten, shake out your arms and do one more set.

*If you want to become
the best runner you
can be, start now.
Don't spend the rest
of your life wondering
if you can do it.*

PRISCILLA WELCH

CHAPTER 10

Final Thoughts

MEMBERSHIP IN the Pasadena Pacers has grown almost exponentially in the last five years, but the prevalence of injuries has not and I attribute this to a consciousness we have about keeping ourselves healthy as we run. We are aware of the possibility of injuries so we stay vigilant for the first signs of their causes, and we do the things we know will keep injuries away.

Here are ten ways we have found to keep injuries to a minimum. They are not ranked in any particular order, although in my opinion, number ten is the most important.

1. Stretch before and after
Lengthen and warm muscles. Maximize blood flow. Don't let tight spots take hold.

2. Warm up
Go out easy rather than blasting the first quarter mile. Make sure your legs are ready for what's to come.

3. Add mileage slowly
Stay within the 10% per week guideline for adding total miles, but be careful about increasing the mileage of your weekly long run as well.

4. Choose your routes wisely
Favor well-lit, low-traffic, smooth surfaces over bumpy and rutted places with poor lighting, high traffic and safety concerns.

5. Rest
It's the magic cure for most running injuries, and the best preventive strategy as well.

6. Listen to your body (ward off injuries before they take hold)
Your body will experience telltale signs that appear prior to an injury setting in, such as serious fatigue, imbalances in your gait, unusual soreness. Learn to notice these signs and back off accordingly.

7. Shoes
Wear the right pair and replace it in a timely fashion.

8. Cross-train
Take the time and effort to work out in ways that do not repeatedly stress the same muscle groups as when you run, and strengthen complementary areas.

9. Strong core
Maintain great running form even when you are fatigued by strengthening your core muscles.

10. Run with friends
Transform your experience of running and benefit from the energy of others who are working together for individual achievement and the well-being of all.

INDEX

A

Achilles 43, 48, 51, 52, 53, 62
Achilles stretch 50
Achilles tendinitis 48, 51
Advil 34
Air quality index 79
Aleve 34
Ankle injuries 46
Antibiotic ointment 58
Arch supports 33, 36, 43, 45
Arthritis 26, 40, 41

B

Back problems 58, 62
Blisters 56, 58, 59
Bunions 57
Bursa 40, 42, 48

C

Calf sleeves 45
Chiropractor 39
ChiRunning 62, 99
Cold, running in 72, 73
Cold weather gear 72
Collapsing arch 52
Compression socks 45
Crime 80
Cross-training 26, 37, 93, 94, 95, 96, 164
Cycling 55, 95

D

Dehydration 76
Dogs 70, 80, 81
Duct tape 59

E

Electrolyte 77
Elliptical trainer 95
Endorphins 22, 66

F

Fatigue 23, 35, 62, 76, 94, 95, 116, 164
Femur 32, 40, 41
Flat feet 46, 106, 110
Foam roller 33, 35
Foot injuries 50
Frostbite 73
Fuel belt 56

G

Glide 59, 65
Gluteals 31, 96
Group running 23, 31

H

Hamstring 35, 43, 62, 61, 76
Heat 76
Heel lift 33, 51, 60, 63
Higdon, Hal 80

Hip muscles 31, 32, 33, 37

Hydration 76, 77, 78

Hydration belt 77, 78

Hydrogen peroxide 58

Hyperthermia 76

Hypothermia 73, 76

I

Ibuprofen 34, 51

Ice 33, 34, 42, 43, 45, 50, 51, 53, 55, 57, 59, 76

Identification 78, 83

Illiotibial band 32, 34

Illiotibial Band Syndrome 29

Insoles 33, 55, 57

K

Knee 29, 30, 31, 32, 33, 37, 39, 40, 41, 42, 43, 44, 45, 50, 54, 63, 95

Knee pain 30, 39

L

Leg injuries 44, 48

M

Mapmyrun.com 71

Metatarsal bone 54

Metatarsalgia 54, 55, 57

Mp3 Phenomenon 67

MRI (magnetic resonance imaging) 44, 55

N

Night splints 52

NSAID (Non-steroidal anti-inflammatory drug) 34, 35, 41, 51, 53

O

Orthotics 33, 36, 43, 45, 53

Osteoarthritis 40, 41

Over-pronating 32, 35, 36

Over-supinate 34

P

Pasadena Marathon 75, 78, 79

Pasadena Pacers 22, 26, 67, 74, 80, 82, 100, 113, 163

Pelvic alignment 37

Physical therapist 39

Plantar fasciitis 50, 52, 53

Pollution, running in 79

Pronating 43

Psoas 31, 37

R

Rest 25, 26, 30, 46, 54, 55, 57, 59, 164

Rollerblading 37, 96

Rowing 96

Runner's high 22, 66, 67

Running barefoot 55, 108

Running boom 21, 22, 23, 108

Running in traffic 67, 68, 79

Running, safety 65

Running shoes 23, 45, 70, 103, 104, 105, 106, 107, 108, 109, 112,

Running shoes, cushioned 40, 110

Running shoes, motion control 110

Running shoes, recycling 112

Running shoes, stability 110

Running shoe stores 59

Running with a group 23, 82

Runtheplanet.com 71

S

Sensory perception 65, 66

Shin splints 44

Short-leg Syndrome 62

Side plank 34

Spenco patches 58

Sprained ankle 34, 37, 46, 48, 49

Strength training 39

Strengthening 37, 41, 49, 53, 61, 96, 115,
    116, 164

Stress fractures 44, 46, 54, 55

Stretching 25, 32, 33, 35, 38, 41, 51, 52, 53, 55,
    57, 59, 61, 113, 115, 116

Stride 30, 36, 45, 50, 62, 100, 105, 116

Supinating 43

Swimming 39, 55, 95, 103

T

Tensor fascia latae 31

The Stick 35

Tibia 31, 40, 41, 44

Traffic, running in 39, 62, 67, 68

U

Ultra-thin shoes 55

USATF (USA Track & Field) 71

Y

Yoga 37, 38, 39

4893922R00094

Printed in Great Britain
by Amazon.co.uk, Ltd.,
Marston Gate.